A Process-Based Approach to CBT

About the Authors

Dr. Michael Svitak, born 1969, studied psychology in Regensburg (Germany) and Reading (UK), receiving his doctorate at the University of Salzburg (Austria) in 1998. Since 2004, he has been head psychologist at the Center for Behavioral Medicine at the Schoen Clinic Bad Staffelstein and also a supervisor and trainer for process-based cognitive behavioral therapy.

Prof. Dr. Stefan G. Hofmann, born 1964, studied psychology in Marburg, receiving his doctorate in 1993. Since 1999, he has been professor of psychology at the Department of Psychological and Brain Sciences at Boston University and has had tenure at Boston University since 2003. Since 2021, he has been Alexander von Humboldt Professor, LOEWE Top Professor, and head of the Translational Clinical Psychology at Philipps University Marburg. His research and work interests are mechanisms of treatment change and emotion regulation, and cultural expressions of psychopathology.

Michael Svitak
Stefan G. Hofmann

A Process-Based Approach to CBT

Understanding and Changing the Dynamics of Psychological Problems

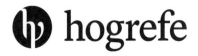

Library of Congress Cataloging in Publication information for the print version of this book is available via the Library of Congress Marc Database under the LC Control Number 2023949436

Library and Archives Canada Cataloguing in Publication

Title: A process-based approach to CBT : understanding and changing the dynamics of psychological problems / Michael Svitak, Stefan G. Hofmann.

Other titles: Prozessbasierte Psychotherapie. English

Names: Svitak, Michael, author. | Hofmann, Stefan G., author.

Description: Translation of: Prozessbasierte Psychotherapie: Individuelle Störungsdynamiken verstehen und verändern. | Includes bibliographical references.

Identifiers: Canadiana (print) 20230558208 | Canadiana (ebook) 20230558216 | ISBN 9780889376281 (softcover) | ISBN 9781616766283 (PDF) | ISBN 9781613346280 (EPUB)

Subjects: LCSH: Cognitive therapy. | LCSH: Psychotherapy. | LCSH: Mental illness—Treatment.

Classification: LCC RC489.C63 S8513 2023 | DDC 616.89/1425—dc23

© 2024 by Hogrefe Publishing

http://www.hogrefe.com

Cover image: © shutterstock.com / optimarc

The present volume is a translation of M. Svitak and S. G. Hofmann, *Prozessbasierte Psychotherapie* (ISBN 978-3-8017-3071-0), published under license from Hogrefe Verlag, Germany. © 2022 by Hogrefe Verlag.

The authors and publisher have made every effort to ensure that the information contained in this text is in accord with the current state of scientific knowledge, recommendations, and practice at the time of publication. In spite of this diligence, errors cannot be completely excluded. Also, due to changing regulations and continuing research, information may become outdated at any point. The authors and publisher disclaim any responsibility for any consequences which may follow from the use of information presented in this book.

Registered trademarks are not noted specifically as such in this publication. The use of descriptive names, registered names, and trademarks does not imply, even in the absence of a specific statement, that such names are exempt from the relevant protective laws and regulations and therefore free for general use.

PUBLISHING OFFICES

USA: Hogrefe Publishing Corporation, 44 Merrimac St., Suite 207, Newburyport, MA 01950
Phone (978) 255 3700; E-mail customersupport@hogrefe.com

EUROPE: Hogrefe Publishing GmbH, Merkelstr. 3, 37085 Göttingen, Germany
Phone +49 551 99950-0, Fax +49 551 99950-111; E-mail publishing@hogrefe.com

SALES & DISTRIBUTION

USA: Hogrefe Publishing, Customer Services Department,
30 Amberwood Parkway, Ashland, OH 44805
Phone (800) 228-3749, Fax (419) 281-6883; E-mail customersupport@hogrefe.com

UK: Hogrefe Publishing, c/o Marston Book Services Ltd., 160 Eastern Ave., Milton Park,
Abingdon, OX14 4SB
Phone +44 1235 465577, Fax +44 1235 465556; E-mail direct.orders@marston.co.uk

EUROPE: Hogrefe Publishing, Merkelstr. 3, 37085 Göttingen, Germany
Phone +49 551 99950-0, Fax +49 551 99950-111; E-mail publishing@hogrefe.com

OTHER OFFICES

CANADA: Hogrefe Publishing, 82 Laird Drive, East York, Ontario, M4G 3V1

SWITZERLAND: Hogrefe Publishing, Länggass-Strasse 76, 3012 Bern

No part of this book may be reproduced, stored in a retrieval system or transmitted, in any form or by any means, electronic, mechanical, photocopying, microfilming, recording or otherwise, without written permission from the publisher.

Printed and bound in the USA

ISBN 978-0-88937-628-1 (print) · ISBN 978-1-61676-628-3 (PDF) · ISBN 978-1-61334-628-0 (EPUB)
https://doi.org/10.1027/00628-000

Contents

Foreword by Steven C. Hayes 5

Preface 9

Part I Theoretical Foundations

1 Limitations of Diagnosis-Oriented Psychotherapy 13
1.1 Inadequate Conceptualization of Mental Disorders 13
1.2 Complexity and Dynamics of Mental Disorders 14
1.3 Somatic or Latent Disease Model 15
1.4 Applying Linear Thinking to Complex Systems 16
1.5 Heterogeneity of Diagnoses 18
1.6 Nomothetic Versus Ideographic Explanatory Models 19

2 Theoretical Foundations of Process-Based Approach 21
2.1 Process Level: Space Between Narrative and Diagnosis 21
2.2 Processes: The Origins of Behavior Therapy 23
2.3 Allostasis Model 27
2.4 Psychopathology: Complex Dynamic Networks 28
2.4.1 Time Dimension: Variability Over Time Makes Processes Visible 30
2.4.2 Stable Networks: Homogeneous and Strongly Interconnected Elements 32
2.4.3 Development of Mental Disorders From a Network Perspective 33
2.4.4 Transdiagnostic Network Structures 34
2.5 Psychotherapy: Network Changes at the Process Level 36
2.6 From Sick to Healthy: Overcoming Network States 37
2.7 Typical Process Patterns Causing Psychopathology and Suffering 39
2.7.1 Unproductive Process Loops 40
2.7.2 Missing Balancing Feedback Loops 42
2.7.3 Maladaptive Inhibitory Control Processes 43
2.7.4 Bottlenecks and Tipping Points 44
2.7.5 Core Dimensions With Strong Influence on the Overall System 45
2.7.6 The Inaccessability of Positive Emotional Network Structures 46
2.7.7 Difficulties in Emotional Processing Hinder Learning Processes 46
2.8 Examples of Process-Based Disorder Models 47
2.8.1 Comorbidity of Depression and Anxiety 47
2.8.2 Prolonged Grief Disorder 48

3 Process-Based Models of Mental Disorders 51
3.1 Diathesis-Stress Model 52
3.2 Process-Based Diathesis Model 52
3.3 Process-Based Complex Network Model 55

Contents

4 Core Processes of Psychopathology 57
4.1 External Demands or Stressors 57
4.2 Vulnerability Mechanisms 58
4.2.1 Neurophysiological Level 59
4.2.2 Emotional Level. 61
4.2.3 Behavioral Level 69
4.2.4 Cognitive Level. 72
4.2.5 Level of the Self. 76
4.2.6 Attachment and Relationship Level. 77
4.2.7 Specific Constructs 78
4.3 Response Mechanisms. 79
4.3.1 Behavioral Core Processes. 80
4.3.2 Cognitive Core Processes 82
4.3.3 Emotional Core Processes 84
4.3.4 Motivational Core Processes. 85
4.3.5 Social and Interpersonal Processes 88

5 Psychotherapy From a Process-Based Perspective 91
5.1 Core Processes of Psychotherapy 91
5.2 Process-Based Therapeutic Stance 92
5.2.1 Capturing Complexity With All Perceptual Channels. 93
5.2.2 Collaborative Empiricism 93
5.2.3 Informed Consent. 93
5.2.4 The Therapist as a Person 94
5.2.5 Dealing With Errors and Uncertainties 95
5.2.6 Flexibility and Loyalty to the Common Treatment Rationale 95
5.3 Evaluation of Adaptivity Based on Evolutionary Principles 96
5.3.1 Variability 97
5.3.2 Selection. 97
5.3.3 Retention 98
5.3.4 Context 98
5.3.5 Physiological and Social/Cultural Level of Analysis 99
5.3.6 Application of the Principles of Evolution in the Psychotherapeutic Context 99

Part II Applying the Process-Based Approach in Practice

6 Phases of Process-Based Psychotherapy. 103
Phase 1: Multidimensional Diagnostic of Relevant Processes. 104
Phase 2: Core Processes: Creating a Process-Based Diathesis Model. 106
Phase 3: Developing an Individual Process-Based Complex Network Model 107
Phase 4: Defining Therapy Goals and Evaluating Readiness for Change 108
Phase 5: Selecting and Implementing Interventions. 108
Phase 6: Monitoring and Reevaluation of the Perturbation Model 108

7 Phase 1: Multidimensional Diagnostics of Relevant Processes. 111
7.1 Spontaneously Reported Symptomatology: Recognizing Processes 112

7.2	Specified Exploration of Conditional Factors at the Process Level	113
7.2.1	Exploring External Coping Demands (Threats)	113
7.2.2	Understanding Internal Coping Demands	115
7.2.3	Identifying Vulnerability Mechanisms	116
7.2.4	Identifying Problematic Response Mechanisms	117
7.2.5	Understanding the Effects and Consequences	118
7.3	Process-Oriented Functional Analyses	119
7.3.1	Selecting Relevant Problematic Situations	119
7.3.2	Process-Based Functional Analysis	119
7.4	Longitudinal Analysis of Symptom Development (Life Chart)	120
7.5	Treatment History	124
7.6	Including External Perspectives	124
7.7	Context Analysis: Protective Factors and Risk Factors	125
7.8	Process-Oriented Assessment of Psychopathology	126
7.9	Using Traditional Diagnostic Methods to Identify Relevant Processes	127
7.9.1	Established Test Procedures	127
7.9.2	Questionnaires for Specific Process-Oriented Constructs	127
7.9.3	Neuropsychological Testing and Biofeedback Methods	128
7.10	Further Process-Orientated Methods: Self-Observation and Visualization Instruments	128
7.10.1	Recording Emotion Regulation Processes	129
7.10.2	Recording Cognitive Processes	134
7.10.3	Recording Behavioral Processes	135
7.10.4	Recording of Somatic Processes	137
8	**Phase 2: Developing a Process-Based Diathesis Model**	139
9	**Phase 3: Developing an Individual Process-Based Complex Network Model**	141
9.1	Practical Procedure for Developing a Complex Network Model	141
9.2	Evaluating the Adaptivity of Network Patterns Using the Extended Evolutionary Metamodel	144
9.2.1	Variability	144
9.2.2	Selection	144
9.2.3	Retention	145
9.2.4	Context	145
9.3	Practical Example	148
9.3.1	Individual Process-Based Complex Network Model	149
9.3.2	Complexity	149
9.3.3	Core Dimensions	150
9.3.4	Accessing Adaptivity	150
10	**Phase 4: Defining Therapy Goals and Creating Readiness for Change**	151
10.1	Defining Global Therapy Goals	151
10.2	Defining Targets of Change at a Process Level	152
10.3	Capturing Readiness for Change	153
10.3.1	Determining the Current Phase of Motivation	153

10.3.2	Cost-Benefit Analysis for Change	154
10.3.3	Determining the Type and Duration of Motivation Required for Change	155
10.3.4	Subjective Prognosis of Success Limits Change	159
11	**Phase 5: Selecting and Implementing Interventions**	161
11.1	Selecting Interventions	161
11.1.1	Defining Effective Dimensions to Target	161
11.1.2	Selecting Interventions to Change Core Processes	162
11.1.3	Planning the Sequence of Interventions	164
11.1.4	Weaken the Maladaptive Network or Strengthen the Coping Network?	165
11.2	Implementing Interventions	165
12	**Phase 6: Monitoring Change and Constant Reevaluation**	167
12.1	Negative Versus Positively Oriented Monitors	168
12.2	Critical Thresholds and Bottlenecks in Therapy	168
12.3	Criteria for Ending Therapy	168
13	**Outlook**	171
References		175
Appendix: Worksheets 1–18		185
Notes on Supplementary Materials		213

Foreword

Why a Process-Based Approach Is the Next Logical Step in CBT

A process-based vision is not new to cognitive behavioral therapy (CBT), but our field has been through so many years of narrowing, caused in part by our own success, that today it can feel as though it is entering the field orthogonally rather than as a historical foundation. An evidence-based approach to psychological intervention began with the task of applying well established principles to the problems of an individual, but it was not long before the central task came to be to diagnose a problem based on signs and symptoms, to categorize these under a specific mental disorder label, and to apply a manualized set of interventions aimed at reducing those signs and symptoms. CBT was spectacularly successful in that task, and that approach helped CBT prosper world-wide. But a sense of stagnation has now arrived, due in part to the galling fact that our effect sizes are not increasing (Hayes, Hofmann, & Ciarrochi, 2023). We need a new way forward.

A process-based approach returns our field to the difficult but exciting task of modeling the complex interplay of affect, cognition, attention, sense of self, motivation, and overt behavior, along with processes in the sociocultural and biophysiological domains, in order to understand why problems arise and persist and how to resolve client problems and promote greater prosperity. Instead of the fruitless pursuit of latent mental diseases, our field is moving towards a new vision in which it is the task of the CBT clinician, and all evidence-based clinicians, to answer this question: "What core biopsychosocial processes should be targeted with this client given this goal in this situation, and how can they most efficiently and effectively be changed?" (Hofmann & Hayes, 2019, p. 38).

The book you have in your hands takes a sober look at the situation and draws on the now large body of basic and applied knowledge regarding process of change, from basic science to third-wave methods in CBT, and applies it to the radically "transdiagnostic" task of answering the key "what," "why," and "how" questions that have always been part of our professional and scientific journey. Why did this problem develop in the first place? What are the goals of the client and what is needed to initiate change? How will change become self-amplifying or be maintained?

This well-written book is not a cookbook of methods, nor it is theoretical tome. It is a practical process-based road map that describes in a step-by-step fashion how to take a process-based approach to CBT, and how to so deeply understand the dynamic of your clients' psychological problems that they can be changed in a systematic fashion that is both strategically sensible and empirically sound.

While traditional evidence-based therapy often employs a nomothetic approach, aiming to generalize from a sample population to individual cases, a process-based approach is idionomic in nature, focusing on the unique characteristics of individual clients but then generalizing them as warranted to nomothetic principles, provided always that the clarity of the individual is thereby increased or at least not compromised. A client is never treated as an "error term" in this approach, nor in this volume. Each unique person is still unique, and a process-based approach sets as its goal that the person will be seen even more clearly and heard even more thoroughly by the analytic steps taken.

That is not mere rhetoric. You will sense as you use the methods this book contains that they bring you as a provider closer to the idiosyncratic details that often get overlooked when we focus on latent disease entities. You will better understand your clients and the options you have to create progress will be more illuminated.

A process-based approach moves practitioners away from a static, linear, pauci-variate model of psychopathology to one that is dynamic and network-based. A process-based approach accommodates complex models of causality, such as feedback loops and dynamic systems, which capture the nonlinear and multicausal nature of psychological phenomena. This approach enhances our understanding of why treatment works when it does and sets the stage for more targeted, kernelized, individualized therapeutic strategies.

This process-based approach recognizes and enriches the strengths of CBT. Svitak and Hofmann are not saying "let's discard our CBT methods." Instead, they are saying "let's understand why our interventions work, for whom, and under what circumstances."

Pursuing a process-based approach is akin to training to be a master chef who knows not just the recipe but also the intricate interactions between ingredients – the subtleties that transform a dish from good to great. It seeks not to replace CBT but to evolve it, to move from a focus on what we should do in therapy, to how and why we should do it, in a way that is attuned to the individual complexities of each client. It is an invitation to be more nuanced, more flexible, and, ultimately, more effective in our practice.

This well-written book lays out the problems of traditional diagnosis and its excessive focus on a nomothetic search for latent diseases, and instead proposes a more idiographic, complex dynamic network approach to psychological difficulties. This shift is not an abstract academic matter – it is an urgent call to action and attention by researcher and practitioners alike. The subpar remission rates in intention-to-treat samples highlight a daunting truth: We are only partially effective in our therapeutic endeavors.

As network thinking is initially explored by the authors it becomes evident that it matters how we conceptualize and analyze client problems, and their predisposing, contextual, sustaining, and protective or positive factors. The authors detail a system of understanding and tracking the major known processes of change, and how they might be impacted by the core processes of psychotherapy.

English readers might be surprised to find that a forward looking and very well-known German psychotherapist, Klaus Grawe (1995), long ago laid out a vision of a scientifically based psychotherapy that focused on relevant processes of change rather than on diagnoses and therapeutic procedures. Details of his theory have not been well validated but his work makes it easier to understand how a process-oriented approach can indeed provide an umbrella for the systematic application of evidence-based methods that modify the processes establish and maintain a pathological network. It also explains why the German psychological community has been particularly welcoming to a process-based approach and is assuming a leadership role worldwide in this area.

A strength of this volume is the detailed way that these core ideas are linked to phases of process-based psychotherapy, from recognizing processes and exploring their determinates, to creating a process-oriented functional analysis and repeatedly assessing client progress. This is a practical volume that has already gone through the hard test of application in systems of care. When the dynamics of a case are clear, a rational kernel-based intervention plan can be uniquely constructed and targeted toward client needs, and an iterative virtuous cycle of monitored steps towards goal attainment can ensue.

In the latter parts of the book, the focus on practical application, assessment tools, and real-life examples offers a seamless bridge from theory to practice. Therapists are not just offered abstract concepts but actionable steps, forms, measures, and strategies to bring the process-based approach to life within the therapy room and system of care.

We have to acknowledge that while meta-analyses already show that taking a more personalized approach produces small but significant therapeutic gains (Nye et al., 2023), a lot remains to be done empirically. But this approach is more a model of how to apply existing knowledge than a radically new set of proposals disconnected from our existing research base and therapy traditions. You can still be you in a process-based approach and the methods that matter can still be used. What is different is your ability to do so is guided by process-based evidence that has been there all along, unseen because of our excessive latent disease focus.

Each era of psychotherapy brings with it new insights, tools, and challenges. The shift towards a process-based approach, as articulated by Svitak and Hofmann, is not just the next phase of this journey but shows every sign of being a transformative leap. It holds the promise of deeper understanding, more effective interventions, and the potential to touch and transform countless lives.

Steven C. Hayes, PhD
Foundation Professor of Psychology Emeritus
University of Nevada, Reno, NV

Preface

If you can add up, that is often enough to deal with most basic requirements in everyday life. If the requirements become more complex, the concept of adding up becomes limited. Then it's helpful when you learn to multiply and divide to understand and deal with more complex demands. Suddenly, previously complicated tasks seem easy. The incomprehensible takes on a logic that helps you to keep track of more complex tasks and to find solutions.

From this point of view, we psychotherapists have become very good at adding up, but we reach our limits with the high degree of complexity we are confronted with in treating our clients, especially when mental disorders do not only occur once but recur or manifest themselves in combination with other disorders. The remission rate in intention-to-treat samples is usually below 50 % (Cuijpers et al., 2010; Spijker et al., 2013). (Intention-to-treat means that the data of all clients who were previously intended to be treated are also evaluated afterwards. This ensures that the data of clients who do not benefit from a treatment and drop out are also evaluated.) We could blame the 50 % failure rate on our clients, but perhaps our current models of mental disorders limit the effects of psychotherapy because we cannot grasp the complexity with our existing models. Perhaps our models of psychological suffering do not adequately represent the complexity and dynamics of mental problems, or perhaps we are focusing on the wrong aspects. Where do we find the complexity and dynamics of mental disorders if they are not sufficiently to be found in the current causal models of disorders? This book is all about focusing on the level of relevant processes, instead of looking at symptoms and syndromes that are often merely a result of these underlying processes. This helps us understand the dynamic interactions of multidimensional processes clients are suffering from in more depth and opens up perspectives for change that are concealed on a symptom level.

From the Symptom Level to the Process Level

Normally, cognitive, emotional, behavioral, motivational, and interactional processes work well together so a person can cope with ongoing demands. In a healthy state, we are as unaware of these coordinated background processes of the mental adaptation apparatus as we are of the work of our PC's operating system. We only become aware of them when the initiated psychological processes aren't successful and either lead into processing loops that generate more and more information or result in processes working against each other. We perceive these underlying adaptation processes gone rogue as a kind of psychological strain, draining psychological energy until we fear the mental system goes haywire or collapses. When clients are asked what percentage of their mental energy is being absorbed by unsuccessful inner processing attempts to solve their problems, many respond: "Over 90 %. And it feels like it's getting more all the time."

From a process-based perspective, mental disorders are the result of these multidimensional adaptation processes gone wrong, so that a formerly healthy state transforms into a system state experienced as stressful (Hayes et al., 2015). So, while we are used to focusing on the level of symptoms, the dynamics and complexity of the regulation process is found at a level "below" the symptoms: at the level of processes, where processes interact with each other to react to demands to the adaptation apparatus. The visible symptom level is merely the result of interacting processes.

Process-based approaches (Borsboom et al., 2011; Hayes et al., 2015; Hayes & Andrews, 2020; Hayes & Hofmann, 2018a, 2018b, 2020; McNally, 2016; Robinaugh et al., 2016) have the potential to add promising new dimensions to our understanding of the complexity and dynamics of mental disorders. They view psychopathology as dynamic networks in which interacting processes are responsible for maintaining pathological system states (Hofmann et al., 2016).

In the first part of the book, we present the most important theoretical foundations of the process-based approach and explain what a process-based view means for our conception of mental disorders and their treatment. In the second part of the book, we describe the practical application – step by step through the phases of a therapy. We hope this approach will inspire your work with clients as it did us. After we spent some time considering the implication of a more process-based approach, we began to look at mental disorders more through a process lens. This helped us to look beyond the content of the disorder and identify the relevant underlying process patterns. This has broadened our understanding of mental disorders and revealed opportunities for change that would have remained hidden through a diagnosis-oriented perspective.

Part I

Theoretical Foundations

1
Limitations of Diagnosis-Oriented Psychotherapy

1.1 Inadequate Conceptualization of Mental Disorders

Why bother with mental processes? Is it not enough to know the diagnosis and select the right evidence-based therapy? It works in somatic medicine, does it not? With the establishment of psychotherapy in health care, paradigms of somatic medicine have been applied to conceptualize mental problems. According to the latent disease concept of somatic medicine, it should be possible to identify diseases based on symptoms that differ in etiology, course, and responsiveness to treatments. This model promises to greatly simplify therapy and allow therapists to provide effective treatment even without an individualized understanding of the individual processes involved. Similar to the approach in somatic medicine, a prescribed treatment is derived from the diagnosis. This is almost standardized for all clients. The goal of this approach is that treatments can be offered in a disorder-specific, manualized, evidence-based, and guideline-driven manner. The associated hope is to treat according to a prescribed set of measures for each definable mental illness, thereby simplifying and improving treatment (Hofmann et al., 2016). As a result of this development, the *Diagnostic and Statistical Manual of Mental Disorders* (5th ed.; *DSM-5*; American Psychiatric Association, 2013) now lists approximately 350 disorders for which more than 270 treatment manuals exist, and their efficacy is more or less well supported by outcome studies (Hofmann & Hayes, 2018). In many studies, the effectiveness and superiority of cognitive behavioral therapy (CBT) approaches over other methods could thus be demonstrated (Heidenreich & Michalak, 2013).

In the textbook or in the guidelines, this makes psychotherapy sound simple, almost like a cookbook. Depression can be determined by asking about nine symptoms using a checklist. If at least five of the nine symptoms are reported, the client can receive the diagnosis. But does this represent the psychotherapeutic reality? Are mental disorders so easy to categorize? Does it really make sense to define an arbitrary combination of five of the nine possible symptoms as depression? Why aren't psychotherapies more effective if the psychotherapists treating them only have to reach for the right manual? The psychotherapeutic reality is actually more complex, dynamic, and individualized than the *DSM* and *ICD* (*International Statistical Classification of Diseases and Related Health Problems* of the World Health Organization, WHO) classification systems and the guidelines derived from them suggest (Deacon, 2013; Hayes, Hofmann, & Ciarrochi, 2020; Hofmann et al., 2016; McNally, 2016; Nelson et al., 2017). Neglecting this complexity and dynamic leads to limiting treatment outcomes on a practical level, which alienates psychotherapists and clients alike. Moreover, ignoring complexity and dynamics on a theoretical level hinders the advancement of psychotherapy because existing model conceptions that are disconnected from reality treads on the spot, instead of creating more refined models (Hofmann & Hayes, 2018; McHugh et al., 2009).

For the practitioner, the question also arises to what extent it is useful to know the more than 270 treatment manuals for the more than 350 *DSM-5* categories if in individual cases it is unclear which comorbid disorder should be treated in which order with which therapy components. Especially in the outclient setting, the flood of disorder-specific approaches can overwhelm therapists and lead to the unsystematic application of different therapy components (Harvey et al., 2009). As a solution many therapists resort to a one size fits all approach, in which one treatment method is applied to all clients. Instead of using the evidence-based procedure designed for a specific disorder, a preferred method of treatment is used (Harvey et al., 2009). This is reflected in statements such as "I normally work according to acceptance and commitment therapy (ACT), which seems to suit me" or "I work eclectically, based on my personal opinion."

The limitations of the current heterogeneous and overlapping diagnostic groups derived from the assessment of subjective client data have also been recognized by the American National Institute for Mental Health (NIMH). It initiated a comprehensive, multidisciplinary project over ten years ago to identify diagnostic groups based on measurable biological and behavioral process dimensions. Known as the Research Domain Criteria (RDoC) initiative, this project aims to diagnose mental disorders using clinical neuroscience methods rather than subjective symptom descriptions. This will involve, for example, electrophysiological and imaging techniques that map neurological structures or functions, genetic analyses, and standardized tests to study learning processes under laboratory conditions. As a result, mental disorders should be traced to core biological and behavioral dimensions (Insel et al., 2010). The dimensional nature would solve the problem of cut-off boundaries and better map the fluid transitions between mental health and mental illness. The hope is that valid structural or functional disease entities can be found at this biological level of analysis to replace the current categories. Although the project does not yet have direct consequences for changes to the existing *DSM* categories, it demonstrates that a paradigm shift should occur and that future models of mental disorders must be conceptualized dimensionally at a process level rather than categorically at a symptom level (Hofmann & Hayes, 2018) so that further development of concepts of mental disorders and their treatments is not hindered (Hayes, Hofmann, & Ciarrochi, 2020).

1.2 Complexity and Dynamics of Mental Disorders

In my practical work (M. S.), in the context of a psychosomatic clinic, singular disorders, as presented in most textbooks, are not only the exception, but virtually nonexistent. The results of the National Comorbidity Survey (Kessler et al., 1994), in which more than 65,000 persons were examined, showed that almost 80 % of the diagnoses were already comorbid disorders; in the case of severe mental illnesses, three or more other disorders were present in 89 % of the cases. The complexity and possible combinations of symptoms in two to three disorders are so great that the supposed simplification provided by a diagnosis-oriented approach is lost. The currently dominant disorder-specific approaches are therefore only suitable for a few exceptional cases.

The results of comorbidity studies also support the low discriminant validity of diagnostic categories (Brown & Barlow, 1992) and that individual disorder components interact with each other at a transdiagnostic level (Harvey et al., 2009). Furthermore, what we see phenotypically at the symptom or diagnostic level has no clear correspondence at the process level. On the one hand, the same processes can be responsible for the development and maintenance of different mental disorders (Fisher et al., 2018; Harvey et al., 2009): A rumination process can maintain a depression, a generalized anxiety disorder, or a somatoform disorder. On the other hand, very many different processes can result in the same diagnostic category (Harvey et al., 2009): The core process behind depression can be a negative self-schema, but it can also be difficulties regulating negative affect, behavioral deficits, or relationship difficulties. The possible combinations of multidimensional, transdiagnostic processes are enormous. This possibility for variation explains, first, the great interindividuality of mental disorders and, second, the great variation in mental health complaints across the life span (Harvey et al., 2009). The assumption that common core processes are responsible for the development and maintenance of different disorders also explains why recorded comorbid mental disorders improve in treatment studies, even if they are not specifically treated (Borkovec et al., 1995; Brown & Barlow, 1992; see also Harvey et al., 2009).

These findings indicate that isolated illnesses as classified in the *DSM* or *ICD* are rare, and thus attention should be focused on core transdiagnostic processes of psychopathology and psychotherapy (Hayes, Hofmann, & Ciarrochi, 2020; Hofmann & Hayes, 2018).

1.3 Somatic or Latent Disease Model

Transferring the diagnosis-oriented approach of somatic medicine to mental illness only makes sense if the individual symptoms are produced – independently of one another – by an underlying disease entity (see left side of Figure 1). For example, a lung tumor produces the symptoms of cough, chest pain, and breathing difficulties. If the disease disappears, the symptoms caused by the disease disappear. This model, which assumes existing disease entities, has been applied to mental illness, although the individual symptoms are usually not independent of each other ("axiom of local independence") and symptoms can persist even if the disease disappears (Hofmann et al., 2016).

The right side of Figure 1, on the other hand, depicts a disease model based on a network understanding: Here, the individual symptoms of disorders interact highly with each other and contribute to overlapping diagnostic categories. The mental disorder *is* the network of interacting symptoms and processes (e.g., rumination process, avoidance behavior, emotional states). The symptoms and the interactions between these processes *are* already the pathology to be treated and do not indicate an underlying disease, as assumed in the "latent disease" model of somatic medicine (left side of Figure 1) (Hofmann et al., 2016). According to the network model, mental disorders can be viewed as a dynamic network or complex system. The elements of this *psychopathological system* are interact-

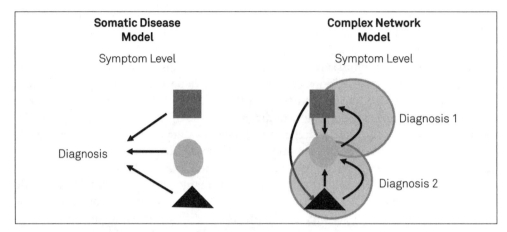

Figure 1. Somatic disease model (left) vs. complex network understanding (right). The symbols in the middle represent different symptoms.

ing processes at the cognitive, emotional, somatic, and behavioral levels. Because of these multidimensional interactions, the psychopathological system, similar to other complex systems (e.g., the weather), cannot be described with linear or causal models. It is dynamic and nonlinear and thus requires a different approach.

1.4 Applying Linear Thinking to Complex Systems

In everyday life, a relatively linear and causal way of thinking is usually sufficient. I am out of coffee, so I have to buy coffee. If I am hungry, I eat something. If I have a psychological problem, I think about solutions. And that's where it starts to get complex. Thinking can contribute to the solution. But the thoughts can also branch out and reinforce the problem or even create new problems. The pondering can make you feel helpless, and the helplessness can trigger a chain of other feelings, such as inferiority and guilt. As a result of my ruminating, behaviors or relationships may change. The psyche consists of numerous subsystems that are highly interconnected. Such complex systems cannot be represented with linear cause–effect notions. They behave dynamically and nonlinearly.

Understanding complex systems such as mental disorders requires a systemic perspective (McKey, 2019; Meadows, 2008). A system can be described simplistically using three components: It consists of (1) elements (what is seen), (2) connections or relationships among these elements, and (3) a function or purpose of the system. The latter can be seen in the effects (see Figure 2).

The system "soccer game" for example has the elements player, ball, goal, and field. The relationships are the actions in the game that occur between the elements and the applied rules affecting the game. The purpose or function is to get the ball into the opponent's goal and at the same time prevent the ball from entering your own goal while adhering to the rules. What is the most important thing if you want to define or understand the system behind a soccer game? If you change the elements (players), it is still a soccer game. However, if you change the relationship patterns, for example, by having oppos-

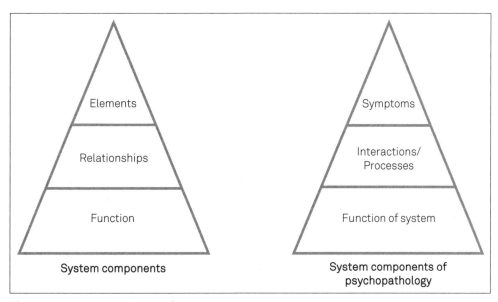

Figure 2.   Psychopathology from a systemic perspective.

ing players pass the ball to each other, the system changes. The impact on the system becomes even stronger if you change the function or purpose. If the purpose is not to touch the ball (avoidance), the system "soccer game" collapses. Although the elements (players) seem to play an important role, the interactions on the process level and the function of the system are by far more important from a systems perspective. In addition, this example is a good illustration of the effects of a system focused on avoidance: Such a soccer game would quickly become unbearable for both players and spectators.

This picture can be transferred to the diagnosis-oriented view of mental disorders, which focuses on the visible symptoms (elements) or the content: We mistake the elements (visible symptoms) for being the decisive thing, but this does not really help us understand the dynamics of the psychopathology involved in mental disorders. It is not the symptom itself – such as negative thinking – that defines psychopathology, but how negative thinking affects mood, behavior, or relationships and how interactions between elements create patterns that cause the individual to suffer. So, the interactions are more important than the elements. Even more defining for a system is the function or purpose. If the elements and the interaction between elements is to "avoid uncertainty," the system will develop into a different state than if the function or purpose is to "grow and learn." Similar to a sports game, the *interactions* between the elements (processes) and the *function* (purpose) are the essential thing to understand the complex system of a mental disorder. Consequently, if we want to change the "mental game" through therapy, we have to influence the game processes and the game purpose – not the elements. That means not changing the thoughts and emotions, but changing the way a person relates to these elements.

This is important in that it is usually the elements of the system that are visible, but the processes can only be experienced through the effects and by recognizing patterns (McKey, 2019). Symptoms are not in general a problem. We all have negative thoughts, we ruminate, have mood dips, or feel inadequate. Only when these symptoms start to interact with each other and cause dynamics that lead to enduring suffering do they become relevant in a clinical sense. But still, it is the dynamic interactions of the processes causing the problems – not the symptoms.

1.5 Heterogeneity of Diagnoses

As clinicians, we have become accustomed to the fact that the diagnosis says little about the reality of the disorder. Two different people diagnosed with major depression may have completely different clinical pictures: One may be completely incapacitated and suicidal and therefore need to be placed in a closed psychiatric ward, while the other may visit a psychotherapeutic practice after work with a relatively inconspicuous outward appearance. At the symptom level, myriad combinations are possible, so that two people with major depression according to *DSM-5* may share only one symptom out of a possible nine. Fried and Nesse (2015) were able to show that if all the subsymptoms of depression are included, 16,400 different symptom profiles are possible. There are 280 depression questionnaires with a variety of different symptoms. The seven most common methods use 52 symptoms, whereas the *DSM-5* system uses only nine symptoms (Dalgleish et al., 2020; Fried, 2015). Even when diagnoses remain the same, there is high phenotypic plasticity between diagnostic categories across the life span.

Sticking to the analogy of a soccer game: The categorial diagnosis of a mental disorder is about as informative as a photo of a soccer match (see Figure 3). At this level of observation, one sees *what* is being played, but not *how* it is being played. The dynamics and complexity of the (game) process are not captured. Moreover, the temporal dimension is not captured by this static snapshot. Looking at the progression of the disorder over time, one perceives how individual aspects of the disorder influence each other. For example, withdrawal behavior can lead to more brooding, and this in turn can increase withdrawal. It is not the individual symptoms that are the problem but the way they reinforce each other and make the sufferer feel helpless. By looking at changes over time, one can infer cause–effect relationships and form hypotheses about processes operating in the background (Gloster & Karekla, 2020).

In a soccer game, a trainer needs to watch a game evolve to see which tactics lead to success and which jeopardize it. On this basis, considerations can be made as to how a team can improve its game: What game processes would have to change in order for the style of play to change? What should the team train on to be more successful? Improving the game and developing competencies of a specific team to become more successful is not possible on the basis of the static information of a snapshot. To make improvements, the coach needs to observe the variations of the game processes, to gain an understanding of the dynamics and functioning of the game. Applied to psychopathology, this means that a snapshot of symptoms is not sufficient to understand the dynamics of the disorder. Only when I understand how cognitive, emotional, and behavioral processes play together to repeatedly create a net of depressive symptoms can I understand and individually address the maintaining conditions of the depressive network.

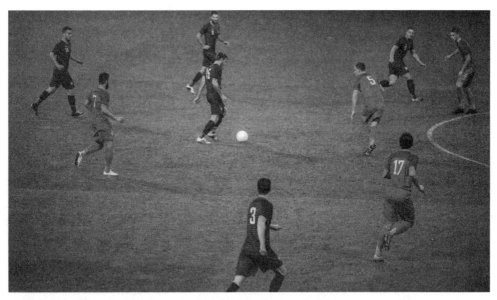

Figure 3. The diagnosis of a mental disorder can be compared to a snapshot of a soccer match. It does not allow any statement about which processes determine the game. The dynamics of the game and how well a team is performing are hidden when you are not able to analyze the interacting processes over time (© iStock.com/simonkr).

1.6 Nomothetic Versus Ideographic Explanatory Models

The oversimplifying diagnostic categories of *DSM* are not only a problem for therapists. Clients, too, often do not recognize themselves in the diagnoses. Sometimes this is experienced as a tug-of-war in which the therapist focuses on disorder-specific factors, whereas for the client, an individual conditioning factor plays a far greater role in causing distress. Although a diagnosis-oriented and manualized approach has set treatment standards and facilitated basic modeling of individual mental disorders (Clark et al., 1997), the emphasis on diagnosis has obscured the view of individual processes relevant to the disorder as well as individual and contextual factors (Hayes, Hofmann, & Ciarrochi, 2020; Hofmann & Hayes, 2018).

The problem arises, among other things, from the fact that clinical research derives most of its knowledge from studying groups and comparing people with and without a diagnosis. It examines how variables differ at a group level, rather than how they behave at an individual level. If it is found that depressed people have lower activity levels compared to nondepressed people, it is reasonable to conclude that depressed people should be activated. On average, this statement is true for the group as a whole, but it is not applicable to a specific person in a specific situation (Hofmann et al., 2016). What is true for the group is far from true for each individual group member. Often, individual group members deviate greatly from the group average. The average shoe size is relatively uninteresting when you want to buy shoes: You do not buy a size that would fit a statistically determined average person, but shoes that fit you.

In contrast to *nomothetic* models, which look for general regularities, *ideographic* models try to explain the individual and particular in each case. Steven Hayes illustrates the difference between ideographic process research and nomothetic research in his lectures with a simple example. When examining typing proficiency at the group level, people who can type very quickly will be proficient and therefore make fewer errors. In contrast, when examined at the individual level, higher typing speed leads to more errors. Both research methods examine the relationship between typing speed and error frequency. However, the results of the two research methods are opposite. It would therefore be wrong to transfer the results of the group study to the individual level and recommend to beginners in a typing course: "Research has shown that people who type quickly make fewer errors. Therefore, type as fast as you can." However, this is exactly the mistake we make when we transfer the results from nomothetic research to individuals (Hofmann, Curtiss & Hayes, 2020).

Ideographic process knowledge is the core of process-based psychotherapy. In ideographic process research, one looks at how variables change in an individual person and how these variables interact with other variables over time at the individual level. This individualized conception also explains how the same processes can result in different disorder categories (Fisher et al., 2018). In one case, worry and thought loops can lead to the development of generalized anxiety disorder. In another case, this derailed cognitive process combined with low self-esteem can promote depression. In a third case, together with increased self-attention to physical symptoms, it may condition a somatoform disorder. However, an exaggerated rumination process can also remain without major consequences. One client who worried constantly reported that this was her way of being close to other people. Worrying, she said, meant that she was well and felt connected to other people. She did not find worrying stressful. In fact, for her, the worrying process had positive effects because it kept her in contact through her caring motive.

These remarks illustrate that the diagnosis-oriented approach primarily considers factors that are supraindividual or represent general effects. The process-based approach, on the other hand, is interested in ideographic processes that are responsible for the emergence and maintenance of psychological distress in a particular person, in a particular context, at a particular time (Hofmann & Hayes, 2018).

2
Theoretical Foundations of Process-Based Approach

This chapter summarizes the main theoretical and empirical foundations that led to the development of the process-based approach in the tradition of cognitive behavioral therapy (CBT). They extend the well-established cognitive behavioral concepts to include insights from complex network theory and empirical findings on transdiagnostic vulnerability and response processes that contribute to the development and maintenance of mental disorders and human suffering. In this regard, the process-based approach does not represent a new school of therapy but rather adopts a different level of observation. Instead of looking at mental disorders on a diagnostic or symptomatic level, it analyzes the processes that contributed to the development of these phenomena. At this level, one can see how individual, dynamic processes influence each other and thereby unfold disorder dynamics. Thus, the focus is on process and network properties that determine whether the interactions form a stable functional system or a pathological network causing an individual to suffer.

2.1 Process Level: Space Between Narrative and Diagnosis

When a person seeks psychotherapeutic treatment, they usually tell a story about their problems and what effects these have on their well-being, work, or private environment. This narrative assembles the perceptible aspects of the experience of a mental disorder from the client's point of view into a plausible story. It usually contains assumptions about causes and causal relationships. "After I got a new boss and the pressure at work increased, I developed sleep disorders, was irritable and depressed, withdrew, was unmotivated and listless," a client might relate in the initial interview. The symptoms are the individual elements of their narrative.

According to current diagnosis-oriented treatment practice, the therapist will extract symptoms from the narrative stream and abstract them to a diagnostic level. According to this logic, for example, the behavior of the new boss is a situational trigger for a depressive illness. Elements of the story, such as sad mood, difficulty concentrating, or sleep disorders, are symptoms of depression according to the *DSM*. This turns the individual, interconnected problems into an illness that requires treatment. Once this is correctly captured, the appropriate guideline or treatment protocol can be selected (Hofmann & Hayes, 2018; Stangier, 2019). This approach makes the complexity manageable.

For a health care system with limited resources, such a mechanistic conception of mental suffering is attractive. It promises a high degree of standardization, quality control, and transferability (Harvey et al., 2009). This approach, simplified in Figure 4, also reflects the development of CBT in recent decades, which has been characterized by attempts to develop structured, disorder-specific, and evidence-based therapies for the mental disorders listed in the *DSM* and *ICD* and to simplify treatment through manualization (see also Figure 5). This approach has been empirically validated by efficacy studies showing that diagnosis-oriented treatment has significant effects (Harvey et al., 2009; Hofmann et al., 2016; Stangier, 2019).

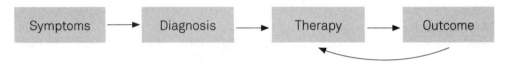

Figure 4. Simple model of evidence-based treatment for mental illness.

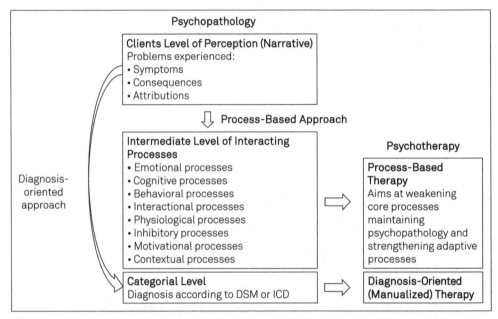

Figure 5. Difference between diagnosis-oriented and process-based approaches. In the diagnosis-oriented approach, the experienced problem constitutes a diagnosis (categorical level). Therapy is carried out according to the treatment guidelines for this diagnosis. In the process-based approach, the focus is on an intermediate level where interacting processes constitute individual psychopathology. Therapeutic strategies are linked to these core processes and target changes at this level.

The process-based approach, on the other hand, focuses – as shown in Figure 5 – on the space between the client's experience and the categorical level of diagnosis. This "intermediate level" is the level of emotion processing, moderating cognitive or behavioral processes as reactions to situational demands on the individual. These processes decide whether the adaptation system stays on top of the incoming demands or fails and causes the individual to suffer from some sort of psychopathology. Thus, from a process-based perspective, analyzing pathology and planning effective treatment starts at this intermediate level (Cramer et al., 2010; Dalgleish et al., 2020; Frank & Davidson, 2014; Harvey et al., 2009; Hayes, Hofmann, & Ciarrochi, 2020; Hofmann & Hayes, 2018).

At this process level are the core processes, now well established empirically across disorders that underlie psychopathology (Dalgleish et al., 2020; Harvey et al., 2009; Hofmann & Hayes, 2018). Sections 4.2 and 4.3 on vulnerability and response mechanisms describe these in more detail. In clinical process research, these vulnerability and response processes mediate and moderate the development, maintenance, and change of psychopathology (Frank & Davidson, 2014; Hayes & Hofmann, 2020).

From a process-based perspective, the goal is not so much to cure "underlying" diseases but to promote processes that enable adaptive and flexible coping with demands the individual is confronted with (Hayes & Hofmann, 2020). The approach focuses on the interstitial space depicted in Figure 5 by analyzing the interacting processes that contribute to the emergence or consolidation of pathological network linkages (Cramer et al., 2010; Hayes et al., 2015; Stangier, 2019). Based on process analyses, interventions are selected that weaken or disrupt system-relevant pathological network processes (e.g., dysfunctional attentional focus) while promoting helpful system activity (e.g., establishing feedback loops) (Dalgleish, et al., 2020; Hayes et al., 2015, 2018). At its core, adaptive responses are always about flexibility with respect to the process dimensions listed in Figure 5 to enable long-term adaptation (Bonanno et al., 2004; Papa et al., 2018).

2.2 Processes: The Origins of Behavior Therapy

The process-based approach does not represent a new school of therapy. Rather, it extends our knowledge about cognitive behavioral theories through the knowledge about processes gained from psychotherapy research over the years. In doing so, the approach integrates modeling ideas from complex network theory and focuses on underlying processes that prevent people from disengaging from a pathological network of distressing feelings, unproductive thoughts, and behavior patterns (Hayes et al., 2015; Hayes & Hofmann, 2020; Hofmann et al., 2016; Hofmann & Hayes, 2018; Stangier, 2019).

The process-based perspective is therefore not new and, in a sense, takes cognitive behavior therapy back to its roots of functional analysis. Behavior therapy at its core has been adiagnostic from the beginning, examining *individual* learning processes that explained both *normal* and *pathological* behavior (Harvey et al., 2009; Kanfer et al., 2006). Gradually, psychological behavioral research integrated more and more system levels broadening the focus to cognitive, emotional, motivational, physiological, and interpersonal processes into its analysis of conditioning factors. From the behavioral research perspective, the focus was strictly on the processes behind visible behavior. Early behavior therapists understood very early on that individual response patterns are linked and automated through classical conditioning and that downstream reinforcing (operant) processes are able to strengthen maladaptive linkages (Dixon & Rehfeldt, 2018; Harvey et al., 2009). From this perspective, the goal of psychotherapy is to disengage established, rigid, but maladaptive linkages (between a trigger and a response) and to develop more adaptive linkages (between a response and a consequence or consequence) that are aligned with target states (Hayes et al., 2018).

The pioneers of behavior therapy still depicted the emergence of problematic behavior in a linear process model (see Figure 6). The SORKC scheme includes situational triggers (S), vulnerability mechanisms (O), problematic ways of reacting (R), and downstream, maintaining contingencies (K) and reinforcer processes or consequences (C). This behavioral therapy model still represents the therapeutic rationale today. In principle, it is already based on a multidimensional diathesis model, but it is still relatively linear. It primarily takes into account conditional factors intrinsic to the disorder that lead to a problematic reaction. Situational conditions usually represent triggers. Feedback processes are limited to the operant effect of consequences on the problematic response (Kanfer et al., 2006).

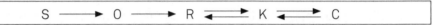

Figure 6. Relatively linear conception of the development of a mental disorder according to the SORKC scheme, supplemented by arrows indicating causal relationships (→) and feedback processes (←).

These linear ideas continue to shape our understanding of the development and maintenance of mental disorders today. However, it is too simplistic to read the SORKC schema from left to right and assume that causal relationships move along this axis. Psychopathology is not static but dynamic, multimodal, and interconnected. We are therefore not dealing with a single response but with a released, self-perpetuating network of response patterns that trigger continuous feedback processes at all system levels.

The interactions between the individual process dimensions (cognitive, emotional reactions, etc.) can be illustrated with the help of connecting arrows. The resulting diagram provides an overview of which process dimensions interact with each other and thus form a kind of "force field." The SORKC model shown in Figure 7 contains a number of process-level interactions drawn in as examples. Thicker arrows indicate strong influence, and circular arrows indicate self-reinforcing processes (Hayes et al., 2015; Hofmann et al., 2016). Activation does not proceed from left to right but follows individual response patterns, which can also proceed from right to left or oscillate between two elements like a pinball. For example, an anxiety-provoking situation (S) leads to avoidance behavior (R) due to vulnerability factors (O), but avoidance behavior also creates new anxiety-provoking situations (S) and reinforces vulnerability factors (O) such as distress intolerance. Individual process dimensions can also be self-reinforcing. This can be the case, for example, when a cognitive activity creates more and more cognitive activity, avoidance leads to more and more avoidance, or negative feelings lead to more negative feelings (see the round arrows in Figure 7). In the "unfolded" SORKC schema shown in Figure 7, the processual information is "in the arrows" which run between the system levels (cognitive, emotional, behavioral, somatic, and interactional levels) (Hofmann et al., 2016). Finally, interactions can occur across systems, such that emotional activity influences relationship regulation or alters context (Hayes et al., 2015).

In Figure 8, the hypothetical interactions between underlying process dimensions are traced to illustrate the multidimensional interactivity at a process level. It shows that the reaction is not as linear as the SORKC model suggests, with a starting point left with an

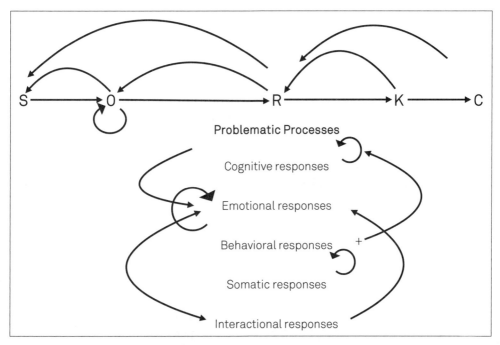

Figure 7. SORKC scheme, where interactions between individual process dimensions are shown with the help of arrows. The thickness of the arrows represents the strength of the connection. Feedback processes are essential but also self-reinforcing processes, where the arrow leads back to the output.

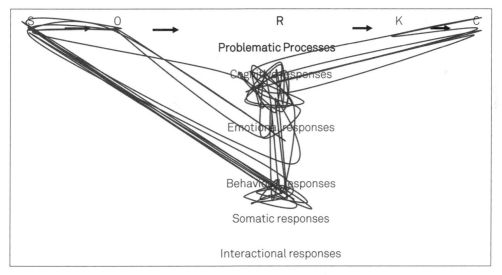

Figure 8. SORKC models showing underlying activation patterns of interacting processes.

eliciting situational trigger (S) interacting with vulnerability factors (O) producing a problematic response that is in some way reinforced. Tracing interactions at the process level reveals individual activation patterns or a map of process network. If certain elements are strongly connected, the lines become stronger. This makes process paths and important nodes visible. Circular patterns also become apparent in this way and indicate vicious circles. The example in Figure 8 shows a lot of activity evolving around the cognitive–emotional responses, suggesting self-perpetuating vicious circles between emotional and cognitive processes and a strong interaction between interactional processes and situational triggers, implying that the interactional response somehow creates new stress-evoking triggers. The figure thus shows a hypothetical map of linkages, or networks, for one individual in a specific situation. Another individual with similar symptoms may show completely different process activity and patterns. Such network maps can also be computed in real terms by taking longitudinal measures of each process dimension and continuously computing individual-level statistical measures of interconnectedness (Hayes & Andrews, 2020).

If we look at the SORKC model from these dynamic points of view, it becomes clear that the superordinate process components (S–O–R–K–C) do not represent a linear sequence of completed process steps. And it is not the content of the cognitive responses or the specific emotion exhibited but the *interactions* – the lines between the content – that create reinforcing dynamics within the system. These interactions are nonlinear and multidimensional (Hayes et al., 2015; Hayes & Andrews, 2020). How they play out is individualized: For example, depending on predisposing factors, negative reinforcement through avoidance might generate strong network dynamics in person X, while having a small effect in person Y. This dynamic could, under certain circumstances, significantly maintain an addiction in person X, while no pathological network structure develops in person Y. The complex network notion attempting to visualize the process activity "brings to life" the SORKC scheme and in a way makes its dynamics visible.

The process-based approach thus focuses on this processual information. It analyzes how cognitive, emotional, and behavioral processes dynamically influence each other and thus form a pathological network of reaction patterns. It "fans out" the SORKC schema and focuses on what happens "in the space" between the S–O–R–K–C elements. At the same time, it does not limit mental disorder to an isolated diagnosis but expands the view across disorders to include the network of process linkages that constitute the entire psychopathology (Hofmann & Hayes, 2018).

When we draw a model of psychological disorder, we often focus on the elements that constitute the components of the model (often the text in the "boxes"). From a process-based perspective, however, more attention should be paid not to these "boxes," i.e., the individual elements of disorder, but to the connections and interrelationships (the connecting arrows) between them. Such a view is initially unfamiliar: The relevant information about the emergence and maintenance of the pathological pattern is not in the text but in the connecting lines or arrows, which vary in thickness depending on the strength of the connection and indicate the corresponding direction of action (Hayes et al., 2015). For example, a depressed client's disorder model includes the element "negative self-evaluation." One would automatically presume that this negative self-appraisal is an element of the depressive disorder and work on helping the client reduce his negative appraisal of himself. However, this is jumping to conclusions. In the process-based approach it makes a difference if the negative self-appraisal is self-perpetuating or reinforces other depressive symptoms, visualized through arrows leading from negative self-appraisal to, for example, negative mood swings, inactivity, rumination, and sleep disturbances. In this case, reducing negative self-appraisal should weaken the depressive network. This may not always be the case. The negative self-appraisal may be the result of other depressive processes. The arrows would lead to the negative self-appraisal. In this case it would take more sense influencing these core processes because this would also halt negative self-appraisal. In some cases, negative self-appraisal may only be weakly interconnected or not a part of the depressive network at all. In this case it may not make any sense in addressing it in therapy for this particular depressed person.

Although dynamic process models are not yet common in psychotherapy, we very often encounter process models in everyday life: They form the basis for weather forecasting. With the help of such models, meteorologists can use the data to detect an approaching hurricane. However, the interaction of wind speed, air pressure, and wind movements visualized by the model does not indicate an underlying weather disease called "hurricane" but represents the multidimensional, complex system we describe as a hurricane. A process-based view of mental disorders follows a similar idea, by analyzing the interactions between multidimensional psychological processes to explain the occurrence and maintenance of process patterns that cause an individual to suffer. The goal is to eventually "visualize" mental disorders in a similar way based on data-generated models, so that it can be inferred that, for example, an "emotional tornado" is in the making (see Chapter 13: Outlook).

2.3 Allostasis Model

Allostasis (Greek: *allo*=variable, *stase*=stable; achieving stability through change) describes a process by which the body maintains stability in demanding situations through physical and psychological reactions or returns to the initial state after a shock. The allostasis concept sees complex, dynamic, and variable adaptive responses at the physical and psychological levels as essential. McEwen (2003), for example, was able to demonstrate the particular influence of social stress on the stress axis (hypothalamic–pituitary–adrenal axis) in the form of the release of cortisol and catecholamines. In this context, expectations, anticipation, and evaluation of demanding situations play a central role in the regulation of the subordinate system levels. The allostatic model thus helps to explain stability through variability of complex systems and accounts for the strong interconnectedness of neurological, psychological, and social processes (McEwen, 2003; Sterling, 2004).

An adaptive network maintains a dynamic tension between stability and variability, thereby forming a relative balance of these two states. These stable patterns in a network are also called "attractor states" or "attractors." The forces between the attractors form a stable equilibrium. When the network is shaken, this allostatic equilibrium is restored by an activation of attractors or by inhibitory processes that create system coherence. Network shocks are absorbed by the overall system, and the network returns to its preferred stable state. That is, a stable network resists change.

Psychotherapy attempts to destabilize an unfavorable network structure (e.g., a network of depressive symptoms) and to establish a new, more positive and flexible network structure with the help of new links. However, this requires a structural change in the existing network structure. Thus, a change from one network structure to another requires a transformation through a series of states of relative stability and variability and a shift in attractor states. A depressed client in whom negative thoughts and feelings are consistent with withdrawal behaviors and negative future expectations cannot seamlessly shift from this state to a state of confidence and self-efficacy. The existing depressive network initially competes with the potentially new network structure. Change is therefore often ruptural, alternating with periods of stagnation or relapse into old network states. This is sometimes observable as sudden improvement in therapy ("sudden gains") or sudden decompensation (Hayes et al., 2015; Hofmann et al., 2016).

The allostasis model is interesting for process-based psychotherapy because it explains the importance of multimodal variability at the process level for maintaining a stable healthy state. Doing nothing or putting the brakes on self-regulatory processes (avoidance) leads to a loss of variability and stability. Healthy regulatory processes are characterized by continuous, fine-tuned, flexible adaptation processes. Disorders at this level, which prevent adaptation, can cause psychopathological conditions. Paradoxically, variability is the basis for stability, and conversely, rigidity leads to system instability (Carver, 2004).

2.4 Psychopathology: Complex Dynamic Networks

In the context of systems and network theories, mental disorders – but also mental health – can be thought of as a force field of interacting processes in which the individual elements are in permanent interaction. The result is a dynamic complex network in which emotional, cognitive, behavioral, physiological, and interactional response patterns interact with prior schemas and modes to form a neural network structure (Hayes et al., 2015). In this process, the processes of the network form a self-regulatory equilibrium that always returns to its original state when shocked, unless the forces and changes require reorganization. The shape of this network is determined by the process patterns, i.e., by how strongly individual processes are interconnected. Mental disorders, as we currently define them, are thus sections of a process or activity pattern in a complex network in which maladaptive processes determine network activity.

Network theory is a branch of mathematics that deals with connections between objects or elements. It helps to visualize complex processes and has been used to describe various complex phenomena (e.g., ecological systems, weather systems, computer systems, and social systems). A network consists of "nodes" (elements) and "edges" – links or associations between the nodes, which are represented as lines (see Figure 9).

In a weighted network, the strength of the association between two elements is represented by a Pearson correlation and by the thickness of the connecting line. In this way, the significance of individual elements – or in our case process dimensions – can be calculated. Interrelationships at the process level thus become visible. Central elements are those whose activity spreads to large parts of the network. They usually have many connections to other elements of the network and thus develop a leverage effect. In a social network, a central element would be a person who has a large influence on many other members.

Complex networks exhibit specific structures or topologies with a typical cluster of activity. Applied to psychopathology, various research groups have been able to visualize individual process interactions as complex network models for various disorders, includ-

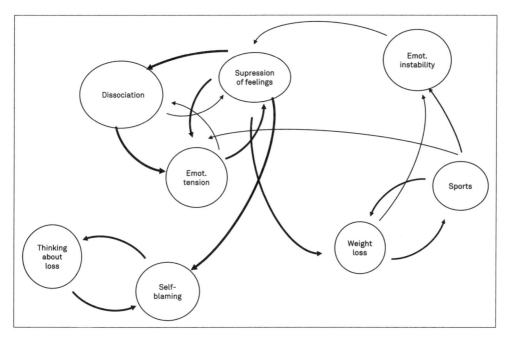

Figure 9. Exemplary pathological network of a client with depression, a dissociative disorder, and an eating disorder with different strong connecting lines.

ing depression (Hayes et al., 2015), complicated grief (Robinaugh et al., 2016), generalized anxiety disorder (Barthel et al., 2020), and posttraumatic stress disorder (PTSD) (McNally et al., 2015; see also Bringmann et al., 2013; Hofmann et al., 2016). More detailed examples will be discussed in Section 2.8.

Network theories help us apply insights of chaos theory to psychopathological phenomena. Chaos theory is a branch of nonlinear dynamics and deals with orders in special dynamic systems, where interactions lead to effects and their temporal development appearing unpredictable, although the underlying equations are deterministic. Wave motions in the ocean follow an order but are still not exactly predictable. Similarly with psychopathology from the perspective of network theory, we can explain how certain symptoms arise, we just cannot predict with certainty when symptoms will occur and to what degree. The model concept of dynamical systems helps to describe nonlinear, dynamic, and transformational phenomena.

It is typical of dynamic networks that they strive to achieve a certain equilibrium. Resilience would be such a stable state, in which a person stabilizes again and again despite shocks. However, in the case of more severe disorders, the system may pass a critical point ("tipping point") and then tips over into a new state, possibly causing the individual to suffer. The stable structure breaks down, the network cannot stabilize again on its own, and a state experienced as pathological or distressing sets in. These clients cannot understand why they have broken down. They report that they have always experienced themselves as robust and stable and that up to now, even stressful life events have had little effect on them. All of a sudden, however, a certain event caused them to "topple over," and since then they seem to get stuck in a state of instability and psychological distress. In this new state, they are irritable, depressed, lack self-confidence, and feel ineffective. The same is true in reverse. A chronic pathological network state can be destabilized and transformed to form of a new more adaptive network structure (Hayes et al., 2015; Hofmann et al., 2016). This is the case when in the context of therapy, a trauma network consisting of the elements of hyperarousal, intrusions, and experiential avoidance loses stability through exposures and the promotion of adaptive emotion regulation strategies, and a more adaptive network structure establishes itself as a new system state. These clients may wonder why the same world that seemed so threatening suddenly feels secure.

This networked view enables the construction of individual complex network models of mental disorders (Borsboom, 2017; Borsboom & Cramer, 2013; McNally, 2016; see also Hofmann et al., 2016). A mental disorder is the sum of network connections whose multimodal network structure generates mental distress (Hofmann et al., 2016). From this perspective, a stressful life event does not trigger a depression that causes the familiar symptoms (Guze, 1992). Rather, the event sets in motion multilayered, interacting processes and counter-processes whose network structure fulfills the criteria of depression (Borsboom et al., 2011).

2.4.1 Time Dimension: Variability Over Time Makes Processes Visible

Through a categorical classification, psychiatric diagnoses give the impression of a relatively stable entity. However, when symptomatology is analyzed intraindividually and longitudinally over hours, days, weeks, or years, it can be seen to be subject to many fluctuations (Molenaar, 2004; Watson, 2004). Inherent in these fluctuations is information about processes underlying the disorder. It is not the variability between individuals that is crucial (nomothetic approach) but the variability within an individual over time. Through adding the temporal dimension, clues about individual processes involved in the development and maintenance of psychopathology become visible. The unit of time – from a few minutes up to decades – determines the degree of resolution. If you look at the entire life span, superordinate influencing factors of the context become visible. Figure 10 shows how a 44-year-old client plotted the development of psychological complaints over her life span. Expressions in the upper third (7–10) indicate severe constraints and high levels of suffering. In this way, the Life Chart reveals rough patterns and typical contextual variables: This client reacted to new life demands like moving out and starting university or becoming a mother with an increase in psychological distress.

If, on the other hand, short sequences of minutes to hours are analyzed, a view of microprocesses is obtained. Figure 11 shows a section of a trauma network. A detailed analysis of the few minutes in which intrusions occur reveals the interrelationships depicted here between the process dimensions involved in the maintenance of these intrusions. In this brief sequence, specific triggers spontaneously and reflexively trigger intrusive memories. As a result, the client responds with attempts at suppressing memories. These paradoxically backfire and produce an increase in intrusions and an increase in hyperarousal. This leads to further attempts to control the emergence of further memories at a cognitive level. The self-reinforcing cycle between intrusive memories, suppression attempts, and hyperarousal is established and leads to further consolidation of symptomatology. In this example, the goal of therapy is to interrupt these self-reinforcing network

Theoretical Foundations of Process-Based Approach 31

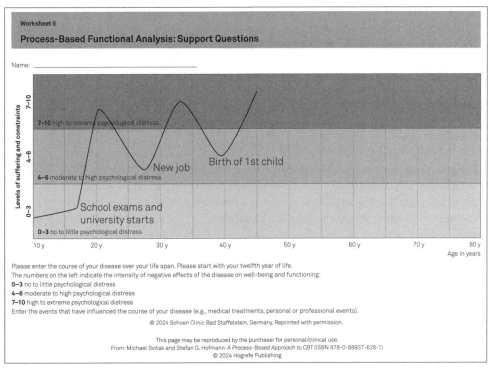

Figure 10. Example of a progression of mental health complaints over the life span (Life Chart). Blank version available in Worksheet 6.

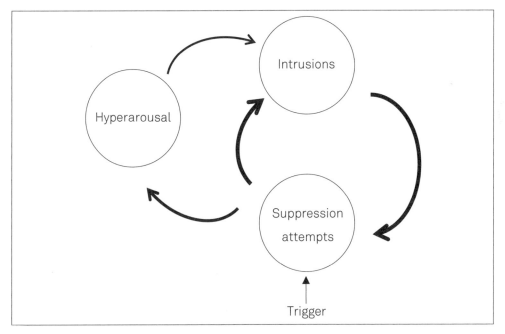

Figure 11. Section of a trauma network describing visualizing the processes maintaining intrusions. The arrows show that the suppression attempts fuel further intrusions and contribute to hyperarousal.

links, which can be recognized as circular thick arrows. The starting point could be preventing the suppression attempts through confrontation methods and emotionally reappraising the memories (McNally et al., 2015).

2.4.2 Stable Networks: Homogeneous and Strongly Interconnected Elements

Once a network has established itself at the process level, this state becomes relatively stable and thus resistant to change. Resistance to change depends on the extent of interconnectedness (connectivity) and homogeneity of the system elements involved. Networks that consist of many homogeneous elements and are at the same time highly interconnected show a tendency toward bistability, i.e., they are either healthy or pathological. From a network perspective, resilience is understood as how quickly a system recovers from destabilization and resumes its initial structure. Less interconnected networks, on the other hand, change more gradually and slowly (Hofmann et al., 2016; Scheffer et al., 2012; see Figure 12, left-hand side).

The resistance to change of once established networks is noticeable in therapy through the reaction to change impulses. Homogeneous and strongly interconnected systems are more stable than less interconnected, heterogeneous networks (see Figure 12, right-hand side). If one tries to unsettle such very stable systems, at first nothing happens. On the contrary, often an irritating strong resistance to change may be felt that sometimes makes

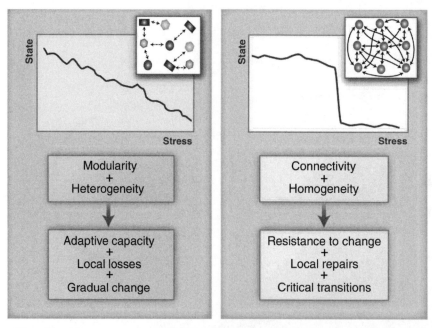

Figure 12. Homogeneous and strongly interconnected networks lead to rupture-like changes. If the elements are more isolated (modularity) and heterogeneous, changes tend to occur gradually. Reprinted with permission from "Anticipating critical transitions" by M. Scheffer and colleagues,, 2012. *Science, 338*, p. 344. © American Association for the Advancement of Science.

therapists wonder whether the help-seeking person really wants to change. It is as if the client is blocking off helpful interventions. This resistance may result in a therapist backing off too quickly, although the increasing resistance may be a sign that the therapy is approaching a significant turning point. Resistance under a network perspective signals progress and requires maintaining the course and waiting until the unsettling state exceeds a threshold that often provokes sudden, ruptural changes in the network structure. Chronic depressive disorders often consist of such homogeneous and strongly interconnected elements, such as a negative view of oneself and the world, negative affect, and negative attention bias. The homogeneity and interconnectedness is like a strong magnet holding the system stable and resisting changes in the network structure. The resulting resistance in therapy should not be interpreted as intentional defensiveness or lack of motivation. The depressive state is more of a nutshell, shielding off external attempts to destabilize the network. A network view therefore helps to distinguish between the strength or resilience of the pathological network and the motivation of the person concerned.

2.4.3 Development of Mental Disorders From a Network Perspective

The characteristics of the networks also influence the onset of mental disorders. Figure 13 illustrates different trajectories in the development of a mental disorder (after Nelson et al., 2017). These well-known patterns of onset depicted in Figure 13 cannot be explained by the static, linear disease models according to *ICD* or *DSM* (Nelson et al., 2017). However, these onset patterns are to be expected from the network perspective and dynamic systems theory. The developmental trajectories shown in Figure 13 can, however, be explained from the network perspective, with the interconnectedness and homogeneity of the network structure determining the way in which psychological disorders develop.

Figure 13A shows the gradual development of a mental disorder in the form of increasing symptomatology in response to multiple stressors. Less homogeneous and interconnected networks (i.e., high modularity and low connectivity of elements) at the process level lead to a gradual development of mental disorders. One client remarked, "It developed insidiously over years. I didn't realize it, that's how slowly it happened." Such a network is like a flexible branch that slowly bends under stress without breaking completely.

Figure 13B shows a sudden crossing of the threshold toward a mental disorder due to a single major stress factor. Viewed from a network perspective, such a development occurs as homogeneous, strongly networked structures suddenly lose their strength and stability from one moment to the next – like a tree trunk that holds up for a long time but suddenly breaks. The disruption begins just as abruptly, as illustrated by one client's statement, "Out of the blue, I broke down emotionally." High connectivity and homogeneity of the elements thus cause the entire network to topple abruptly.

Finally, a (healthy) network can be gradually destabilized by repeated shocks (see Figure 13C): Repeated stressors are accompanied here by increasingly severe and prolonged symptoms. Initially, a rapid recovery is observed; over time, the recovery phases last longer and longer. It can be assumed here that relatively homogeneous and interconnected network structures are gradually destabilized by repeated shocks until the structure gives up

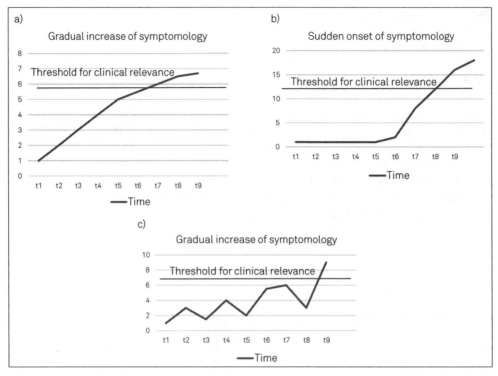

Figure 13. Development of psychological disorders as a reaction to stressors (adapted from Nelson et al., 2017). a) Shows a gradual increase until the threshold is reached and the symptoms become clinically relevant. b) Shows a sudden onset, when the network "snaps" from a nonpathological state into a pathological state. c) Shows repeated stressor events, and the network becomes less and less resilient until the network transforms into a pathological state. *Note.* (Panel A) Gradual deterioration of mental state due to response to stressors. (Panel B) Sudden transition to a psychopathological state triggered by a sudden, highly salient stressor. (Panel C) The development of the mental disorder is already indicated by the increasingly severe responses to stressors and increasingly prolonged periods of recovery. See further explanation in the text.

resistance and enters a pathological state. This is illustrated by the following statement of a client: "I had already taken a bit of a bashing. The last event was the straw that broke the camel's back."

2.4.4 Transdiagnostic Network Structures

Elements of different disorder categories may also be highly interconnected and overlapping. The pathological network shown in Figure 14 illustrates how elements of the depressive network are connected to elements of the generalized anxiety disorder network. There are also elements or processes that may be part of multiple diagnostic categories. Ruminative thinking can be transdiagnostically an important process of depression, generalized anxiety disorder, and posttraumatic stress disorder (PTSD) (Wells, 2009). Alternatively, there are elements that act as a bridge between disorder domains. Social with-

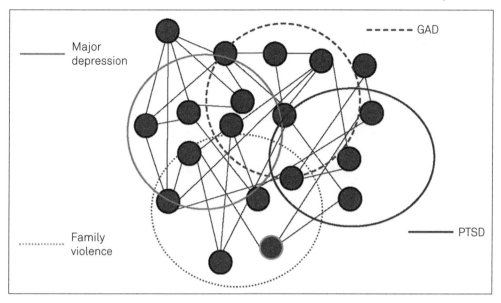

Figure 14. Psychopathology as a transdiagnostic network showing overlapping symptoms between major depression, PTSD, GAD and effects of family violence (adapted from Hayes et al., 2015).

drawal can be such a bridging symptom that on the one hand promotes rumination processes of a generalized anxiety disorder and at the same time activates intrusive memories of a PTSD. Thus, a psychological network is multidimensionally interconnected across disorder boundaries.

The network conception also allows contextual factors to be included in the consideration of psychopathology, rather than being categorized solely as situational triggers (Hayes et al., 2015; Hofmann et al., 2016; Hofmann & Hayes, 2018). Looking at the exemplary pathologic network shown in Figure 14, an external contextual factor such as ongoing family violence may be essential to the persistence of the other problem areas. Focusing on guideline-based treatments for depression, generalized anxiety disorder, or PTSD does not do sufficient justice to the network of interconnected problems. Mapping the network across systems can help individualize hypotheses about what maintains the disorder dynamics in this person and in this situation. Understanding this forms the basis for deciding which processes need to be therapeutically tackled and in what order to transform the pathological network into a more adaptive network. Is it important to stop the violence first? Or does learned helplessness or a negative self-concept in the context of depression prevent ending the violence and therefore need to be addressed first? Or are transdiagnostic processes responsible for the emergence and maintenance of the overall system, so that a change from one process leads to improvement in all problem areas? There is no universal answer for this. What is correct in this case can only be decided by an individual analysis of the transdiagnostic network of elements constituting the pathological state of an individual on the process level.

2.5 Psychotherapy: Network Changes at the Process Level

The research group led by Hayes and colleagues (2015) has very impressively and systematically described the processes involved in both the emergence and the improvement of psychopathology at a process-based network level. Figure 15 provides an example of how a depressive network becomes interconnected and stable through self-reinforcing problematic processes: (Panel A) The depressive (maladaptive) network consists of many connected elements, and the connections are not so strong at the beginning (thin lines). The curved arrows indicate self-reinforcing vicious circles that strengthen the con-

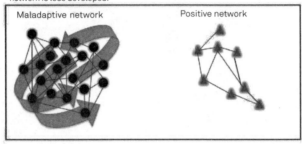

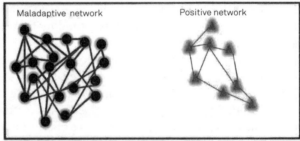

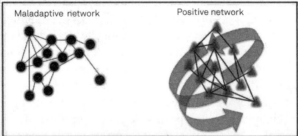

Figure 15. Exemplary representation of a pathological network and the change processes in therapy (Hayes et al., 2015). Reprinted with permission from "Network destabilization and transition in depression: New methods for studying the dynamics of therapeutic change," by A. M. Hayes, C. Yasinski, J. B. Barnes, & C. L. H. Bockting, 2015, *Clinical Psychology Review, 41*, p. 32. © Elsevier.

nections between the elements of depression. This can happen simply by the co-occurrence of symptoms through associative learning, in which the links between depressive symptoms are established and additionally strengthened through operant mechanisms. The result of these self-reinforcing processes is a stable, elaborate network of depressive processes consisting of many interconnected elements. One element activates another until the network has assumed a fixed structure of depressive elements that encloses the individual mentally, emotionally, behaviorally, and physically. A parallel positive network is only weakly formed at this point. In the therapy phase (Panel B) to attempts are made to further establish positive network elements, e.g., through positive activities and helpful relationships. At the same time, links of the maladaptive network are weakened (Panel B: the left network indicates destabilizing links within the maladaptive network). Finally, in the transfer and maintenance phase of therapy (Panel C), self-reinforcing processes are established in the positive network to anchor the person in this more positive mode.

The art of process-based therapy is to recognize and influence the *relevant* process patterns that keep the pathological network stable and the disorder dynamics running. Relevant processes can be recognized by the fact that they are central elements – process elements that are linked to many other elements of the pathological network and thus contribute to the perpetuation of a pathological pattern in the network. A temperament characteristic in the form of a negative affect can be such a central element. Negative affect is usually associated with dysfunctional emotion regulation strategies and a negative attentional focus, while also blocking access to positive affective memories. Thus, this one element of the network has far-reaching negative effects on various subsystems of the adjustment system and makes a relevant contribution to the disorder dynamics (Hayes et al., 2015).

Alternatively, a network element can reinforce itself and thus form a kind of negative energy center. This happens mainly through negative reinforcement, as a result of which, for example, withdrawal leads to further withdrawal, avoidance leads to more and more avoidance, brooding is followed by more and more brooding, and so on. Such unbalanced processes explain the development of vicious circles.

2.6 From Sick to Healthy: Overcoming Network States

From this network perspective, psychotherapy attempts to disrupt a pathological network structure and move the system across a critical threshold (tipping point) into a new, non-pathological network state. The individual elements of a network attract each other differently and thus determine the overall structure and network stability. Therefore, to move from one network state to the next, resistance must be overcome. As described earlier, this can be a gradual process. In many mental disorders, however, we are confronted with a tightly connected and very resistant network structure. An anxiety network, among other things, consists of fixed beliefs about being annihilated if it is not possible to avoid the anxiety, a solidified attentional focus on relevant threat signals, automated avoidance impulses, and other mechanisms designed to prevent the feared annihilation. A depressive network from which a sufferer seeks to disengage usually consists of solidified negative beliefs, avoidance, and recursive cognitive processes that render them helpless (Hayes et al., 2015).

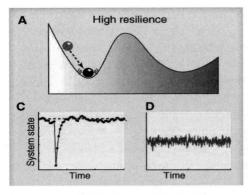 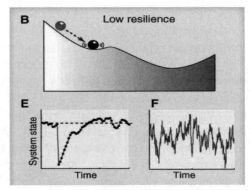

Figure 16. Visualization of the stability of network states. Explanations in the text. Reprinted with permission from "Anticipating critical transitions" by M. Scheffer and colleagues, 2012. *Science, 338*, p. 345. © American Association for the Advancement of Science.

Scheffer and colleagues (2012) and Nelson and colleagues (2017) illustrate the respective network state using an energetic mountain-and-valley model. The mountains and valleys represent different network structures, and the currently experienced state is symbolized by a ball moving through the mountain-and-valley landscape. Stable, resilient systems are represented as deep energetic valleys (see Figure 16A). Here, a great deal of resistance must be overcome to move the ball past a critical point where the network structure re-forms and does not return to its original form. The more established the network is and the more tightly connected elements the network has, the more forces stabilize the network. If the energetic valley ist very deep, the therapist must anticipate a higher level of resistance and the client has to be prepared to invest more energy to overcome this network state and get past the tipping point. That may be difficult to comprehend at first, because clients assume that leaving an unwanted or miserable state to become happy is all downhill. But on the contrary, the pressure and forces that cause the maintenance of the pathological structure become stronger as the ball moves upward. This can be thought of as occurring in a long-standing depression in which the individual elements of the depression are entrenched and tightly interwoven with each other and additionally associated with external contextual factors. One client described this entrenched, multimodal pervasiveness of a network state as follows, "Everything in my life is gray, every thought, every feeling, my movements, my memories, my expectations. Every fiber of my existence is saturated with depression. Even my apartment is contaminated by depression, the walls are drenched in negativity." Attempting to overcome this state activates the depressive network at first, so that the established forces of the system work against change. Affected persons then have the impression that they cannot overcome this state, despite their best efforts, or assume that they may just not want it enough.

Less resilient network states are less strongly interconnected, and the links are more unstable. Such states can be overcome by a smaller shock and transferred to a new network state (see Figure 16B). If an initial pathological state is not very resilient, it takes only a small nudge in therapy to change it. Such therapies are comfortable for psychotherapists: With early intervention and available resources, only a small nudge is sufficient to bring about change.

This "tipping" from one state to the next does not happen out of the blue and can even be predicted from the network perspective. The knowledge for this comes from the investigation of complex networks in other disciplines, such as climate research; this investigates how the world climate is brought out of its existing equilibrium by external influencing factors (e.g., CO_2 emissions). Scheffer and colleagues (2012) were also able to demonstrate this "tipping" for mental disorders. Before a network "tips" it exhibits characteristic features that indicate that it has lost resilience. For example, there is slower recovery after network destabilization (see Figure 16E compared to Figure 16C) as well as greater fluctuations (see Figure 16F compared to Figure 16D) in the configuration of individual elements of the network (Scheffer et al., 2012). This can be thought of as shaking the network links. The fluctuations and the fierceness with which the network structure is defended reflect the resilience of the system (Scheffer et al., 2012).

For therapy, it is important to take these network properties into account. Detachment from the force field of an existing pathological network usually leads initially to an increase in symptoms and is usually experienced as unsettling and destabilizing. Anxiety clients are familiar with this condition from exposure treatments when they ask, "I thought the anxiety would go away with therapy, yet it keeps getting worse. Is there a tipping point where the tension eases? Are you sure my anxiety isn't just going to keep increasing until I go crazy?" What clients feel during a confrontation with anxiety is the escalation of symptomatology to the point where the psychological tension experienced as unbearable is at its maximum and the maladaptive network structure is destabilized. Only the destabilization of the network of origin creates space for the formation of a more adaptive network (Hayes et al., 2015). Eating-disorder clients often report during the phase of gaining weight that their eating-disorder thoughts become more intense, the urge to exercise becomes unbearable, or they can no longer tolerate their body image. This destabilization is understandably experienced as unsettling and is often interpreted by clients as an indication that something is going wrong in therapy. If clients are not prepared for this, the increase in unpleasant symptoms and tensions will trigger an avoidance reaction or lead to discontinuation of therapy.

The image of energetic mountains and valleys through which a ball moves is very helpful in psychotherapy and very catchy for clients. They can use this model to describe very precisely where they are at the moment, what is preventing them from getting past certain tipping points in therapy, or what they fear when they overcome the force field of their pathological network. Statements like, "I'm worried I can't take it. The tension is already unbearable. I don't think I can take it anymore, but I know if I get past that point it will get easier with time and there will be no going back" show that clients feel understood by these complex network models.

2.7 Typical Process Patterns Causing Psychopathology and Suffering

How is it that pathological network states develop? What happens at the process level when processes that generate psychopathology gain the upper hand? The processes of a healthy, stable network normally form a self-regulatory equilibrium that always returns to the original state when shaken, unless the forces and changes require reorganization. This occurs at a multimodal level, where emotional, cognitive, behavioral, and physiological response patterns interact with previous schemas and modes to form a neural network structure (Hayes et al., 2015). In the healthy state, these processes generally run "like clockwork" – synchronously and harmoniously and in accordance with desired allostatic target states.

Psychopathology kicks in when the available reaction mechanisms of an individual are not able to find an adequate solution for a demand stressing the system. So, what is happening on a process level the therapist should look out for? First, processes that run unproductively into the void or processes without balancing feedback loops both tend to merge into unregulated vicious circles. Clients are caught in the same thoughts and feelings, unproductively recycling them again and again. Or clients oscillate between two opposing reactions: like elaborating memories and suppressing them at the same time. When this happens, they may be blocking adaptive processing. Other clients get stuck in the attempt to process demands because they fail to get through bottlenecks or over certain thresholds. For example, they are unable to tolerate the intensity of feelings required to successfully cope with a certain situation, leading them to back off from an otherwise adaptive processing attempt. Finally, functional network areas necessary for processing may be inaccessible and impede processing. Hayes and colleagues (2015), in their highly recommended article on network destabilization and transformation, explain how these process phenomena can transform a healthy network into a pathological network state.

What is important from a therapeutic perspective is that these developments at the process level, which can lead to a psychopathological momentum, also work in reverse. From a therapeutic perspective, the aim is to interrupt negative cycles and reaction cascades or help develop functional processes. From a salutogenesis perspective, process properties can be used to initiate positive vicious cycles and reaction cascades that keep a client's healthy network state continuously stable.

The problematic processes that can lead to the development of mental disorders or contribute to their maintenance are explained in more detail in the following sections.

2.7.1 Unproductive Process Loops

In depressive disorders, the aforementioned "running into the void" can be well observed. Although the response to a difficult situation does not work, the affected person repeats the unsuccessful strategy over and over again, making him feel more and more helpless the more often it doesn't work. For example, a depressed person may stay in bed, hoping to have more energy to get up later. Or they may continue to ruminate, although no new insights are gained by ruminating. Still, the process does not end. Clients suffering from anorexia nervosa may continue to lose weight in order to gain more self-worth, although the desired effect fails to materialize. Psychological disorders often emerge when attempts to cope come to nothing and are unproductive. The problem is not the reaction itself (e.g., staying in bed), but that an unproductive process (e.g., waiting for more energy) is repeated, even though the desired result (e.g., more energy) does not occur.

From a network perspective as described by Adele Hayes and colleagues (2015), depressive disorders are characterized by the fact that sufferers have difficulty detaching their attention from negative stimuli and negative emotional states. Affected individuals perceive something negative, repeatedly focus their attention on it, and the process starts all over

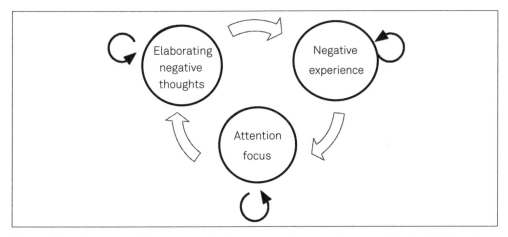

Figure 17. Example of three unproductive process loops at the cognitive level that collectively produce depressiveness.

again. Hayes and colleagues (2015) describe this as an "unproductive processing loop" in which the process goes around in circles. Secondary feelings of helplessness, sadness, or loss of self-esteem are an understandable consequence of unproductive loops. From this perspective, depression is a network state in which the defining elements have rigidly organized around negative valence, low activation, and negative affectivity, and this pattern of activity has become the "home base" through numerous repetitions (Hayes et al., 2015). How unproductive process loops can develop negative momentum is illustrated by the example in Figure 17, where a negative experience through a negative attentional focus combined with a thought elaboration process continues to intensify unchecked.

While unproductive process loops may seem inconspicuous at first, they can transform the complex system in question into a more pathological state with each repetition, or produce rupture-like changes above a critical threshold. Affected individuals describe the latter as a sudden breakdown or crash. In the above example of the depressed person, the negative experience with an unfavorable focus of attention can build up with further depressive elements until, seemingly "suddenly," a suicidal crisis develops. Described from the point of view of one client, this presents itself like this: "In the morning I was still fine. I had spilled my coffee (negative experience). As a result, my mood deteriorated, and I thought about all my problems and injustices (negative attention focus). I thought about my failures (elaboration process) and became unaware of anything around me. After two hours it felt unbearable. And then I didn't want to be there at all." Linear models cannot explain such developments, while they are typical for complex networks.

It is very important to recognize such unproductive, often circular process patterns. They can cause small demands – to which someone reacts with ineffective attempts at a solution – to build up so that a "mosquito becomes an elephant." Again, it is not the symptom that is the problem, but the self-reinforcing pattern. If a symptom increases continuously by 1% per day, then sooner or later this process leads to excess. Instead of brooding or drinking alcohol for an hour a day, the sufferer spends many hours in this self-defeating activity. Once you consider the leverage of unregulated processes you begin to understand why certain processes are unproblematic in one person and escalate in another. It is not the behavior that is the problem, but the unregulated growth process.

This effect becomes even more severe when unproductive processes initiate further unproductive processes at other system levels: unproductive rumination (a self-reinforcing cognitive process) can initiate an equally self-reinforcing negative affect (emotional process). Now, two unproductive process loops are already driving psychopathology. If this ignites a third self-reinforcing process (e.g., avoidance behavior), a multidimensional negative process cascade with cognitive, emotional, and behavioral elements emerges (see Figure 18), which can close into a cycle.

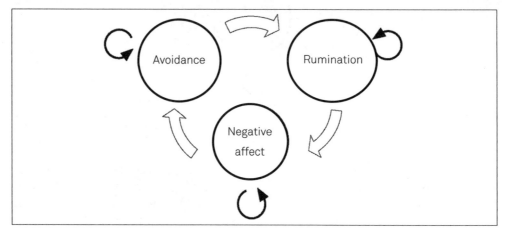

Figure 18. Propagation of self-reinforcing process loops across different system levels. Rumination (cognition) causes negative affect states (emotion) and reinforces inactivity and avoidance (behavior). All three processes create a negative momentum and reinforce each other.

2.7.2 Missing Balancing Feedback Loops

In stable networks, balancing feedback loops are very important to prevent processes from getting out of hand. These are feedback loops that initiate counter-processes or inhibitory processes that balance a system (see Figure 19). An example of this is the hunger-satiety regulation. The hungrier I am, the more I eat. At a certain point, feedback signaling satiety reduces the urge to eat, so a balance between hunger and satiety is maintained. In a regulated system, this coupling of processes and counter-processes is important. If the balancing process is missing or not activated, then a process and its effects may run unabated.

The problem with regulating difficult emotional states is to take into account the time delay between the moment you perceive an unsettling emotional system state and the time it takes until initiated balancing response mechanisms show an effect. Many of our clients with psychological problems have difficulty tolerating this gap between taking action and experiencing an effect. This unsettling time lapse results in people giving up or switching balancing responses too soon or fleeing the situation altogether before any effects of a balancing response show an effect. For example, in a fearful social situation, someone may use a self-soothing affirmation (balancing process) to counteract an increase in fear (reinforcing process). However, the effect of the soothing affirmation will not be immediate and anxious feelings will not suddenly disappear as a result. Fleeing the fearful situation on the other hand shows an immediate effect. This inertia of regu-

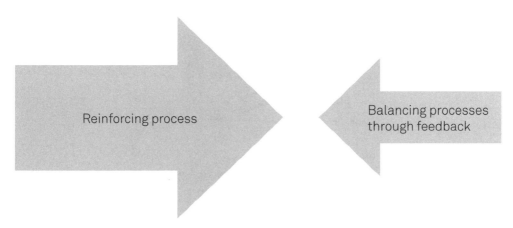

Figure 19. Regulation of systems by balancing feedback loops.

latory systems is sometimes difficult for those affected by mental disorders to withstand, tightening the linkage between fear and avoidance responses and depriving the person of successfully habituating in the situation.

Especially in disorders involving the perception and evaluation of signals (e.g., alexithymia), the lack of balancing feedback loops has a negative impact on the control of regulatory processes (Sheppes & Gross, 2012). In alexithymia, experiencing emotions is flattened, and affected individuals are poor at perceiving and interpreting their feelings. The less accurately feelings are perceived and interpreted, the more difficult it is to match emotion regulation strategies to them. This is similar to people who have lost the sense of hunger and satiety: Normal eating is hindered by the difficulty to perceive and interpret information about hunger and satiety.

Balancing processes serve to continually rebalance and maintain direction even in the face of changes in context. Emotion regulation represents an ongoing process of noticing feelings and responding to them in a way that does not allow one to be "knocked down" by them. To illustrate the ability to deal flexibly with feelings, the term "emotion surfing" is often used in therapy. This image conveys the aspects of emotion assessment and proper timing for successful emotion regulation. The ability to read emotions and predict their course determines whether someone is able to "surf" an emotional wave or whether they will be "submerged" by it. An alexithymic person has difficulties seeing the waves and interpreting their movement and force. His only option is to lie flat on the board and try not to go under. This can be quite frustrating for him, especially when he notices that everyone around him is skillfully progressing on their boards.

2.7.3 Maladaptive Inhibitory Control Processes

In complex systems, response processes can sometimes work against each other and block adaptive regulation (Hayes et al., 2015). In PTSD, unprocessed memories may be activated in one part of the cognitive network in the form of intrusions, and at the same time activated control processes may try to suppress these memories (see Figure 20). Intrusions and inhibitory control processes then block each other. The affected person oscil-

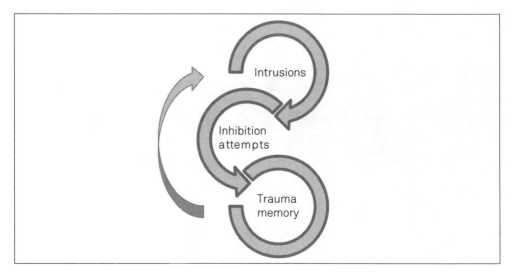

Figure 20. Maladaptive inhibitory processes in dealing with intrusions.

lates between these two states, and the desired processing process gets stuck. This impasse at the process level can initiate further coping attempts. For example, the affected person can decouple from this unpleasant state with the help of dissociations.

These maladaptive inhibitory processes can occur at all system levels. In depressive states, it is conceivable at the neurophysiological level that the combination of hyperactivity of the amygdala and inhibitory cognitive control mechanisms in the dorsolateral-prefrontal cortex may initiate the negative elaboration process already outlined and build up to a manifest depressive state (Frank & Davidson, 2014; Hayes et al., 2015).

2.7.4 Bottlenecks and Tipping Points

In addition to these circular process patterns, process disruptions can occur at certain bottlenecks within the system (McKey, 2019). Usually, the bottlenecks occur because certain consequences of a coping process are not tolerated and therefore avoided. In psychotherapy, vulnerability factors may represent such a limitation in the coping process and condition avoidance. For example, low distress tolerance can be seen as a bottleneck in dealing with intense feelings and lead to the avoidance of emotionally intense states. In some cases, this inability to confront oneself may obstruct dealing with emotionally demanding situations.

This bottleneck in the system can be described using the mountain-and-valley model of Scheffer and colleagues (2012). According to this model, the bottlenecks can be located in the form of thresholds on the mountainside (see Figure 21). Such thresholds can be experienced in the form of anxiety or tension, which increase during the course of therapeutic change until a tipping point is reached. Clients sometimes describe this by saying: "I feel the walls closing in on me. The pressure is mounting. If I could, I would back up and resort to my old strategies that relief the pressure." This progression is readily observable in all exposure-oriented therapies. Initially, this state may feel uncomfort-

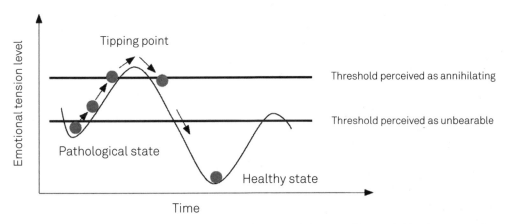

Figure 21. Emotional thresholds as limiting factors of change – illustrated by the mountain-and-valley model (adapted from Scheffer et al., 2012).

able or be experienced in the form of tension. Later, the activated feelings may be experienced as "unbearable" or even "devastating." The limiting constrictions are usually near the tipping point, that is, the point of inflection where the forces of the system are overcome and a new network is formed. In addition to emotional tipping points, cognitive, behavioral, or physiological thresholds can also limit change. For clients in therapy, often the idea of having to think, do, or physically endure something seems unbearable or even devastating. For example, a client with PTSD stated: "Having to think about what happened to me is too much for me. I just cannot allow these thoughts or I'll certainly crack up. The idea of sharing these thoughts with another person is even more unbearable. I'd rather die. And if I don't, my heart will do me the favor and stop beating."

2.7.5 Core Dimensions With Strong Influence on the Overall System

When considering psychopathology at the process level, processes that generate unfavorable leverage in the form of domino effects and reaction cascades on the overall system can be observed time and again. One of the ways this occurs is that these processes limit flexibility at multiple levels. The six elements of the Hexaflex model of acceptance and commitment therapy (ACT; Hayes et al., 1996: Acceptance, Presence, Values, Defusion, Self as Context, Commitment) focus on key core processes that create unfavorable leverage. For example, cognitive fusion affects perception, evaluation, and response selection, and thus regulatory flexibility; experiential avoidance (rather than acceptance) has an equally strong effect on a network's flexibility and therefore produces unfavorable leverage on other regulatory processes.

Healthy regulatory processes are characterized by flexibility. Prerequisites for this are: (1) context sensitivity, i.e., reality-based perception of the world, (2) a flexible repertoire of responses, and (3) feedback loops that feed back information about the effectiveness of the strategy. This requires a target state in the sense of an approximation goal (Bonanno et al., 2004). If one restricts oneself to these prerequisites for regulatory flexibility, a selection of core dimensions emerges that can generate leverage at the process level, depending on how they are expressed. These are compiled in Figure 22.

Negative effects on adaptivity	Positive effects on adaptivity
Avoidance motivation	Approach motivation
Inflexible repertoire	Flexible repertoire
Fusion	Defusion
Illusory processing	Reality-based processing
Lack of feedback loops	Reality-based feedback loops

Figure 22. Important core dimensions with their respective characteristics that can generate positive or negative leverage effects on the adaptivity of systems.

2.7.6 The Inaccessability of Positive Emotional Network Structures

Studies of mental network structures show that depressive disorders are not only associated with a preference for negative network activity but that positive emotional network areas are less accessible and thus more difficult to activate. For example, depressed individuals have difficulty activating positive emotional schemes and memories, which promotes being stuck in the negative network state. This disconnection from positive network regions therefore makes it difficult to form an alternative network or to mentally activate it in the sense of a target state. If positive network regions are more difficult to activate, then the elements of this more helpful network do not act as attractors. In this sense, people suffering from a depressive state have a neglect for positive elements. Thus, regulatory flexibility is severely limited (Hayes et al., 2015). The left part of Figure 23 illustrates this: In the depressed state, initially almost exclusively the depressive network is activated; positive network areas are deactivated (Panel A). Therapy activates positive network elements so that the network expands (Panel B).

2.7.7 Difficulties in Emotional Processing Hinder Learning Processes

The difficulty in accessing the full range of emotional processing described in Section 2.7.6 has a negative impact on learning processes. According to Barlow's (2014) emotion regulation model, functional affect regulation requires the positive affect system. In contrast, one-sided regulation via the negative affect system causes emotion regulation disorders. On the one hand, important emotional context information cannot be processed adequately without the positive affect system, and, even more problematic, helpful expectations, like positive attractor states that control the regulation process are not available. According to Hayes and colleagues (2015), individuals are stuck in a negative state and have no clue as how to escape this negative system.

Theoretical Foundations of Process-Based Approach

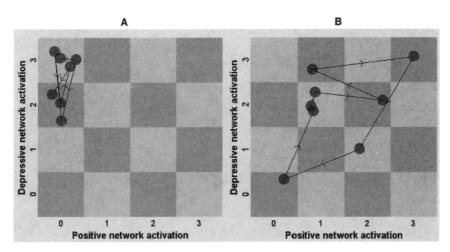

Figure 23. (A) Exclusive negative network activity in the depressed state (blockage of positive network activity) and (B) activation of positive network connections during therapy to create a positive attractor state (taken from Hayes et al., 2015, p. 34).

This narrowing of the emotional network to solely negative elements has direct implications for the flexibility of learning processes. It influences the perception of consequences, restricts expectation formation to negative expectations, and limits the choice of responses (Rief, 2020). In principle, for affected individuals, this is like taking a multiple-choice test where only negative responses are available; helpful responses are not available for selection. Understandably, these repeated unsuccessful attempts at regulation lead to the activation of avoidance patterns, negative self-appraisals, helplessness, and ruminative processes (Hayes et al., 2015).

2.8 Examples of Process-Based Disorder Models

2.8.1 Comorbidity of Depression and Anxiety

We would like to illustrate the advantages of the process-based approach using two process-based disorder models. Figure 24 shows the hypothetical disorder models (in the form of complex networks) of two individuals diagnosed with major depression and comorbid generalized anxiety disorder. At the categorical level, the two clients do not differ. The two networks shown in Figure 24 each have elements of depressive symptoms, anxiety symptoms, and symptoms that function as bridging symptoms between the disorder categories. From a process-based perspective, one can see from the arrows between the elements that for Person A and Person B, however, quite *different* process pathways are responsible for maintaining the disorder dynamics. This example is meant to illustrate that when symptoms and diagnoses are the same, the core processes responsible for maintaining and changing the disorder dynamics are often different. Where starting points for intervention are in the model is indicated by the arrows, not the elements of the network. The disorder models are ideographic, i.e., they map the dynamic disorder events of a single person at a time.

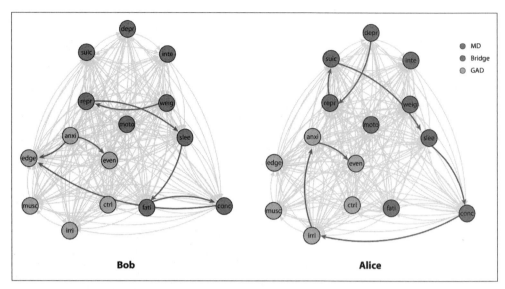

Figure 24. Hypothetical example of complex networks of two individuals with the same diagnoses: major depression and generalized anxiety disorder. The arrows represent causal interactions, the thickness of the arrows depicts the strength of the relationship. Reprinted with permission from "Network analysis: An integrative approach to the structure of psychopathology," by D. Borsboom & A.O.J. Cramer, 2005, *Annual Review of Clinical Psychology, 9*(1), p. 110.

2.8.2 Prolonged Grief Disorder

While Figure 24 shows hypothetical network models, Figure 25 is based on a data-generated, process-based disorder model of a client diagnosed with complicated grief (Robinaugh et al., 2014). For this process-based network model, the statistical measures of association between individual-level subprocesses were continuously calculated. The result represents a representation of the dynamic processes that contribute to the maintenance of the disorder.

In Figure 25, network areas can be identified that show stronger connections and interactions. These patterns of activity in the form of clusters and vicious circles indicate that the elements involved in them maintain the grief network. For example, *emotional pain processing* occupies a very central position in the network and is highly interconnected with other network elements, suggesting that the management of pain experience is very relevant to the maintenance of complicated grief. At the top of the network, the elements of *identity loss*, *emptiness*, and *loneliness* form a self-reinforcing subnetwork, indicating problems in functionally coping with attachment loss. The affected person feels "amputated," "alone," and "empty" without the partner and does not manage to form new attachments. Finally, the elements of *worry about the future*, *denial*, and *numbness of feeling* form a vicious circle (bottom right). These elements interfere with general life coping tasks such as facing day-to-day challenges, overcoming things, and finding new goals.

These network areas around which the disorder dynamics of complicated grief revolve provide therapeutic entry points for coping (see Robinaugh et al., 2014):

1. Network area – "dealing with emotional pain": learning to deal with the emotional pain experienced without falling into avoidance or passive longing;
2. Network area – "attachment regulation": finding ways to process the loss of attachment and reorganizing the internal representation of one's self or identity in order to overcome loneliness and emptiness;
3. Network area – "general life coping": learning to accept the new reality of life and to focus on everyday goals despite being occupied by the feeling of loss.

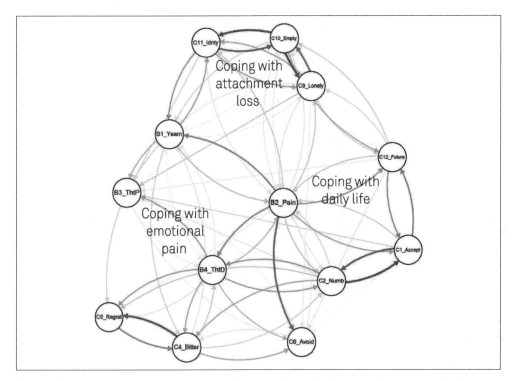

Figure 25. Process-based disease model of complicated grief (adapted from Robinaugh et al., 2014). Explanations in the text.

On the basis of this process-based network model, blockages or competence deficits for the coping process can be elicited and interventions can be precisely tailored to these processes. The affected person does not have to go through a normative mourning process, as suggested by guidelines for coping with grief. The goal is to plan interventions that fade the arrows relevant to this person's individual grief system so that the pathological network dissolves or exerts less pull. The starting points based on such a process analysis can be very individual. It is not the individual processes per se that are dysfunctional; adaptivity can be gauged by the individual impact on a given person's overall network in a given context (Hofmann & Hayes, 2018).

3
Process-Based Models of Mental Disorders

A process-based disorder model is a functional condition model in which the core processes responsible for psychopathology are summarized with their causal relationships. Such a case concept helps to answer the following relevant question: Which processes are responsible for the development and maintenance of the disorder and therefore need to be focused on in therapy in order to bring about change (Jose & Goldfried, 2008)? The basis of the process-based disorder model is a diathesis-stress model focussing on underlying processes (see Section 3.2). According to Macneil and colleagues (2012), such a case concept should include the following elements:

1. *Problem description – understanding individual internal demands:* A problem description goes beyond knowing the overt problem. It describes the multidimensional internal coping demands or stressors in their individual complexity. In the context of the process-based approach, one wants to understand what internal coping demands the person is struggling with. Is it overwhelming emotional pain (emotional level), loss of important bonds (relational level), loss of life goals (motivational level), problem-solving deficits (behavioral level), or social problems (social level)?
2. *Predisposing factors:* According to the diathesis-stress model (see Section 4.1), an external demand or stressor becomes a problem when interacting with predisposing factors that limit coping responses. These predisposing factors are described in detail as vulnerability mechanisms in Section 4.2.
3. *Contextual factors:* This refers to factors that contribute to the development of problems, such as financial, occupational, or family stressors that the individual is struggling with.
4. *Sustaining factors* are the central processes that contribute to the maintenance of existing problems and disorders. These are described in detail in Section 4.3 on response mechanisms. Sustaining factors include aspects such as avoidance behavior, unfavorable attentional focus, and reassurance.
5. *Protective and positive factors*, in the context of the process-based approach, are resources and skills that buffer negative effects, weaken sustaining processes, or promote the development of coping mechanisms.

It is important that the developed disease model will be flexible in integrating new information (Macneil et al., 2012). According to Persons (1989), it should be a continuous process in which relevant information is collected, assessed, reviewed, discarded, summarized, and used to develop new hypotheses for understanding the dynamics of the disorder.

3.1 Diathesis-Stress Model

The diathesis or vulnerability stress model as well as the transactional stress model (Lazarus, 1974) explain on a macrolevel the development of disorders by the fact that stressors interact with existing vulnerability factors. This diathesis or vulnerability establishes the "readiness" for a disorder. However, if the organism responds to the stress factor in an appropriate manner, the development of a disorder can be prevented or mitigated. The effect of the response is also influenced by risk and protective factors. Figure 26 shows a classic diathesis-stress model for an emotional disorder.

The diathesis-stress model forms the basis for process-based conceptions of disorder development and maintenance. Disorders are already explained in the diathesis-stress model in multifactorial, multimodal, cross-diagnostic, and ideographic terms. The model includes factors intrinsic to the disorder as well as contextual factors. Only the interaction of all factors explains the occurrence of a stress reaction and the development of a pathological state. Thus, the diathesis-stress model is very well suited as a starting point for a process-based view of mental disorders.

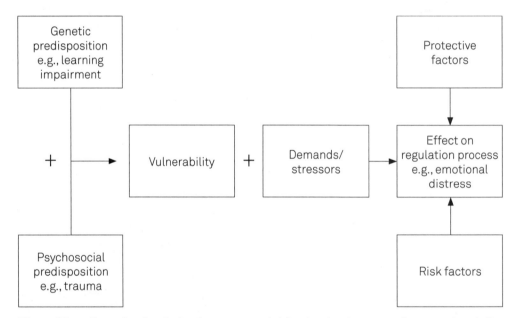

Figure 26. Example of a diathesis-stress model for the development of an emotional disorder.

3.2 Process-Based Diathesis Model

An adaptation of the diathesis-stress model for the process-based approach is the process-based diathesis model. The term "process-based diathesis model" is intended to draw attention to the processes that are involved in the development and maintenance of a person's psychopathology. It explains the occurrence of a mental disorder through the interaction of external coping demands to stressors and the interaction of vulnerability and response mechanisms.

The trigger is a change in context, i.e., an external demand to adapt to. To become a relevant trigger, it commonly has to threaten an individual's central needs or goals in some way. A change in context may threaten physical existence but more often threatens the image of our internalized "self" or attacks core social or personal motives (e.g., for safety, self-efficacy, belonging) or values (e.g., for order, status) (Scherer et al., 2001). This threat prompts an individual to respond in some *way to minimize the threat*.

An unfavorable dynamic begins to develop when *triggering demands* on the organism interact with existing *vulnerability mechanisms* and the system fails to adapt via self-regulatory processes. For example, the developmental task to make new friends after moving to another city only becomes a problem when it encounters vulnerability mechanisms that make making friends difficult (e.g., a strong social insecurity). The organism is confronted with a demand that cannot be handled immediately; thus, a state of tension is created between the desire to make friends and the anxiety triggered by the demand (e.g., fear of rejection). In an attempt to resolve this state of tension and restore balance, *response mechanisms* are activated, such as avoidance mechanisms (helpful in the short term, problematic in the long term), or motivational mechanisms that help to overcome or endure the fear.

These three dimensions: (1) triggering demands/stressors, (2) vulnerability, and (3) response mechanisms are interconnected via continuous feedback loops (Frank & Davidson, 2014). The initiated response either achieves the desired effect and the system is ready for new demands, or the coping attempt is ineffective, in which case the response mechanisms remain activated. The mechanism of interaction of these three dimensions shown in Figure 27 is highly simplified. In reality, new demands continuously hit the system, and

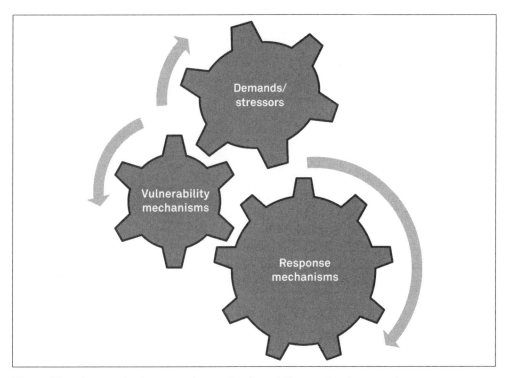

Figure 27. Interaction between demand, vulnerability mechanisms, and response mechanisms.

the system reacts to them. The initial reaction also changes the original stressor, which in turn triggers another reaction cascade. This can be thought of as the image that emerges when standing between two mirrors (Sheppes et al., 2015) – a regulation process never ends, but always produces a result, which is regulated again, and so on.

The process-based diathesis model attempts to capture the processes that are essential for the pathological effects of the interactions between triggering demands, vulnerability mechanisms, and response mechanisms (core processes). Figure 28 shows a simple process-based diathesis model with a selection of core processes (e.g., rumination, low uncertainty tolerance). The focus is on the moderating core processes between demand and impact.

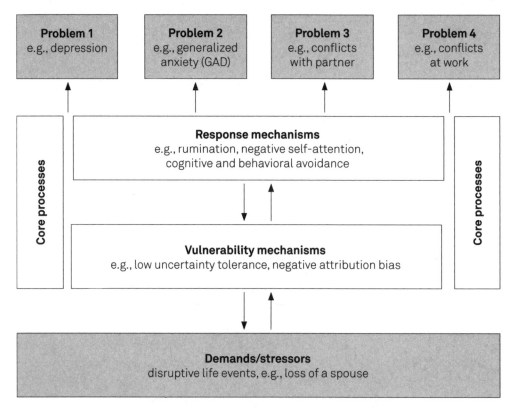

Figure 28. Example of a process-based diathesis model (based on Frank & Davidson, 2014).

From a process-based perspective identifying core processes is a big step in the right direction. However, the process-based diathesis model only tells us something about *which* processes play a role in creating and maintaining psychopathology but not *how* these processes individually interact, causing a system to topple into state that causes the individual to suffer. It is like in music, where it is not enough to know the tones to experience the effect of music, but it is the combination of tones, the rhythm, the spaces in between and intensity that create harmony, disharmony or even different emotional reactions. In order to grasp the underlying, individual process dynamics, a process-based complex network model is derived from analyzing causal relationships between these core processes.

3.3 Process-Based Complex Network Model

In a further step, the core processes captured in the process-based diathesis model and their interactions are now analyzed in more detail to find out which of them significantly cause and maintain psychopathology. The result is an individual process-based complex network model. How to get from core processes to a complex network model is described in detail in Chapter 9. This model maps the individual disorder dynamics at the process level.

Figure 29 shows a schematic representation of an abstract network model illustrating how core vulnerability and response mechanisms interact to create a vicious circle fueling the pathological network. The arrows in the model point to processes that contribute significantly to the maintenance of the pathology. These are the processes that reinforce other problematic processes or form self-reinforcing spirals. In Figure 29, the "problematic response 1" shows a reinforcing dynamic with a vulnerability factor and a further "problematic response 2." The model shows which core process is of significance for maintaining dynamics. From many possible core processes, the problematic response 1 forms a "whirl" or center around which a pathological dynamic is reinforced. Interventions would therefore have to focus on interrupting this driving force.

The complex network model of the disorder thus creates a link between individual processes and derived intervention planning (Nezu et al., 2004; Persons, 1989). It suggests where interventions can begin to interrupt the dynamics of psychopathology. From this point in therapy, a canon of proven, evidence-based therapy methods can be drawn upon, as summarized by the Inter-Organizational Task Force on Cognitive and Behavioral Psychology Doctoral Education (Klepac et al., 2012; see Table 9 in Section 11.1.2).

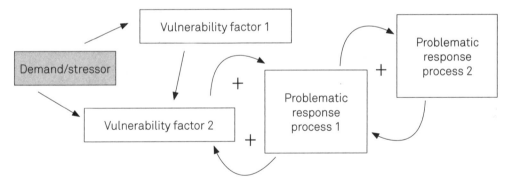

Figure 29. Schematic representation of a simplified process-based network explaining how vulnerability factors interact and initiate problematic responses that are fueled by reinforcing loops.

4
Core Processes of Psychopathology

It is difficult to find something if you do not know what to look out for. The same is true, when looking at the process level and wanting to understand how vulnerability and response processes in coping with triggering demands can contribute to the development of mental disorders. It helps to know what core processes are often linked to psychopathology.

Several groups of researchers (De Houwer et al., 2018; Dixon & Rehfeldt, 2018; Frank & Davidson, 2014; Harvey et al., 2009; Papa et al., 2018) have identified transdiagnostic core processes that are systemically relevant to the emergence of pathological networks. Already, the Hexaflex model of acceptance and commitment therapy (ACT) (Hayes et al., 2009) focuses on six core processes of psychological experience that explain the development of psychopathology. However, in focusing on six specific dimensions, this may narrow the perspective and become dogmatic in the sense that individuality is lost by applying a fixed model. The process-based approach therefore aims to broaden the perspective in relation to further, individual processes that are not derived from a theory, but empirically generated. This open-source model presumes that many relevant processes are first to be discovered.

This chapter provides an overview of the most important empirically proven transdiagnostic processes associated with the development of psychopathology. In doing so, we are guided by the three dimensions of the process-based diathesis model from Figure 27 (see Section 3.2): demands, vulnerability mechanisms, and response mechanisms. For each of these dimensions, we summarize the core processes of psychopathology that have been explored so far. The compilation given below does not exclude the possibility that other processes, which may not yet have been sufficiently researched, exist. Therefore, this is a selection, which can, however, help to sharpen the view of processes.

4.1 External Demands or Stressors

The first component that plays a role in the development of a disorder is an event that triggers coping and adjustment processes. This can be a stressful single event, or it can be enduring stress. From a psychopathological perspective, these are events in the person's world (external or internal) that pose some form of threat and provoke a multimodal response. Such events may represent a real threat to physical or psychological existence, or a threat to important internal representations of self (self-image) or the world (values).

According to self-determination theory (Deci & Ryan, 2008), loss of *self-efficacy* (competence), *autonomy* (voluntariness), and *relatedness* constitute relevant threats. Many everyday events that trouble us can be explained by the disruption of one or more of these three dimensions.

There is a plethora of terms for such an event, such as trigger, event, stressor, or triggering situation, which indicate that this factor comes from outside. For this purpose, we use the general term *external demand* in order to clarify the demand character on the adaptive apparatus. This moves the focus away from the specific trigger situation to the following questions: What individual demands arise from this situation on the various system levels of this person (cognitive, emotional, or behavioral demand)? With which vulnerability factors does the demand interact? Which multidimensional response patterns are activated at the different system levels?

4.2 Vulnerability Mechanisms

Vulnerability mechanisms are conceptualized in behavior therapy as organism variables. They include, in addition to organic or genetic conditions, enduring cognitive or emotional constructs, such as insecurity tolerance or emotional instability, as well as general risk factors that contribute to the maintenance of the client's problems (Frank & Davidson, 2014).

From the perspective of the process-based approach, individual differences exist at the level of vulnerability that determine whether a stressor becomes a problem. Vulnerability mechanisms are key to understanding the client's individual distress. Only through a deep understanding of the client's vulnerability is it possible to develop compassion and coping options that are appropriate for the client.

The term *mechanism* is intended to clarify at this point that it is an applied reaction mechanism in the sense of a predisposition. A change requires a conscious modification by an alternative process that replaces or alters the existing mechanism.

Vulnerability mechanisms have been discussed and researched from the perspective of a wide variety of theoretical concepts, so determining what constitutes a vulnerability factor is often ambiguous. The term is used in so many different ways that it is difficult to narrow it down to a manageable number of relevant vulnerability mechanisms. We understand vulnerability mechanisms as individual differences that make it difficult to cope with demands at the cognitive, emotional, or behavioral level.

We therefore focus on a selection of vulnerability mechanisms that seem relevant to us, drawing on the prior work of Frank and Davidson (2014) and Harvey and colleagues (2009), who systematically captured and assessed core processes across diagnoses. Vulnerability mechanisms at the emotional level, describing individual differences, were additionally described by Hofmann (2019). Table 1 provides an overall overview of the vulnerability mechanisms described in the following sections.

The findings presented often implicitly assume a causality in which vulnerability factors contribute to the development of psychopathology. As explained earlier, this unambiguous causal attribution is invalid in a process-based network view. Vulnerability factors condition psychopathology, but psychopathology in the same way produces vulnerability.

Table 1. Vulnerability mechanisms at different system levels

System level	Vulnerability mechanisms
Neurophysiological level	• Arousal regulation and inhibitory processes • Executive functions • Sleep regulation • Biological components of emotion regulation
Emotional level	• Temperament • Negative affect • Emotional granularity • Alexithymia vs. emotional clarity • Emotional intelligence • Reduced stress tolerance • Affective styles: acceptance • Emotional flexibility
Behavioral level	• Classical conditioning • Operant conditioning • social learning and model learning

Cognitive level	• Memory processes
	• Cognitive fusion
	• Inflexible cognitive schemata
	• Negative schemes
	• Extent of negative thinking:
	  – Dysfunctional attribution bias
	  – Negative control beliefs
	  – Negative problem orientation
	• Metacognitive processes and beliefs
	• Symbolic learning processes: Learning and language

Level of the self	• Inflexibility of the self (including personality disorders) • Negative self-focused attention
Attachment and relationship level	• Attachment representation
Specific constructs	• Regulatory flexibility • Perfectionism

4.2.1 Neurophysiological Level

When dealing with vulnerability factors, one first thinks of organic variables that have a direct influence on regulatory processes. These include tension regulation and inhibitory processes, processes controlling executive functions, basal emotion regulation processes, and sleep regulation.

Arousal Regulation and Inhibitory Processes

People vary in their ability to regulate arousal, calm themselves, or to control behavioral impulses (Harvey et al., 2009). Deficits in these areas inevitably make it difficult to cope appropriately with demands accompanied with a rise of physiological arousal. Furthermore, deficits at this level of coping create new problems, which produce a string of new demands – causing activation spirals that produce more arousal. Increased neurophysiological arousal states are responsible for self-reinforcing loops that negatively affect emotional and cognitive subsystems and impede learning and adaptation processes. If demands experienced as threatening meet an already tense physiological response system, critical thresholds are quickly exceeded so that adaptive coping is no longer possible.

Deficits at this basal level of arousal regulation and impulse control lead to secondary problems at higher system levels, such as attention-deficit/hyperactivity disorder (ADHD; Solanto, 2011), addictive disorders (Batra & Bilke-Hentsch, 2012), PTSD (Henning-Fast & Markowitsch, 2010), panic disorders (Craske & Barlow, 2014), worry (Turk et al., 2005), antisocial behavior, and suicidality (Crowell et al., 2005), and provide the breeding ground for emotion regulation disorders that constitute borderline personality disorder (Linehan et al., 2007).

Executive Functions

Managing a stressful demand requires continuous control and coordination of executive functions: a constant evaluation of the situation, a selection of strategies, a prediction of their effect, a decision in favor of one strategy, and the inhibition of other impulses and constantly modeling the chosen strategy to the context. Thus, executive functions form an important prerequisite of regulatory flexibility (Bonanno et al., 2004). Executive functions are also multidimensional, so that the arousal regulation and inhibitory processes described above have direct effects on executive functions. These deficits in the cognitive-emotional control functions of the frontal brain can be observed particularly in those with ADHD (Solanto, 2011), borderline personality disorder, or PTSD (Aupperle et al., 2012). However, deficits in these executive functions can play a moderating role in all other mental disorders.

Contrary to the previous linear notion of causality between vulnerability factors and mental disorder, the process-based approach assumes reciprocal causality. Impaired cognitive-emotional control capacity may promote anxiety disorders, but anxiety disorders have concomitant negative effects on executive functions (Eysenck et al., 2007). Crucial to the development of pathological network states is the outcome of the interaction between vulnerability factors, triggering situations, contextual factors, and response mechanisms (Frank & Davidson, 2014).

Sleep Regulation

Sleep and emotion regulation are based on similar neurophysiological processes and are thus closely interconnected (Gehrman et al., 2013). In many mental disorders, sleep is disturbed, which is an indicator for problems in the emotion regulation system. Again, no clear causal direction can be discerned between disorders in sleep architecture and emotion regulation disorders, so (1) transdiagnostic processes may be responsible for both, (2) sleep disorders may complicate emotion regulation, or (3) problems with emotion regulation may lead to sleep disorders (Harvey et al., 2009).

Biological Components of Emotion Regulation

The largely genetically determined, biological components of emotion regulation (Scherer, 2009) produce evolutionary bottom-up response patterns to stereotype threat stimuli. Deficits in the dopamine-serotonin regulatory system, for example, can highly disrupt emotion regulation and be involved in the development of bipolar disorder, mania (Miklowitz & Johnson, 2006), or borderline personality disorder (Linehan, 1993). Increased amygdala activation affects emotion regulation and has been shown, for example, in clients with borderline disorders (Herpertz et al., 2001). The likelihood of developing PTSD after trauma also depends on neural structures (Malta et al., 2009). It is not the trauma that determines the extent of impairment, but the interaction between the event being coped with and neurophysiological and psychosocial conditions. If one has good ways of coping with high levels of arousal, as well as a robust emotion regulation system, and if one can rely on one's executive functions, then one will have a better chance to compensate major shocks. If, on the other hand, one has deficits at this level, then one's own response mechanisms are more likely to be overwhelmed and activate emergency or protective responses, such as avoidance reactions or freezing and stalling reflexes (Porges & Lewis, 2010).

4.2.2 Emotional Level

Although emotional reactions and emotional dysregulation are at the core of most mental disorders, they have long been treated stepmotherly, and it has been difficult to even define what emotions are. In the context of psychotherapy, it is generally agreed that emotions are responses to stimuli that are relevant to the self – that is, threatening in some way. From an evolutionary theoretical perspective, situations that threaten physical integrity, loss of resources, or the integrity of the self are relevant to the emotional response system (Ekmann & Friesen, 1982).

Excursus: Emotion Regulation Process

The emotion regulation process is a multidimensional process that combines cognitive, emotional, physiological, and behavioral elements. Individual differences that influence the perception, appraisal, selection, and application of emotion regulation strategies, as well as the ongoing evaluation process of the regulation process, therefore represent an essential vulnerability mechanism. We first discuss this process in more detail, as the mechanisms and potential disruptions of regulation described here can also be applied to other regulation and adaptation processes.

Gross (2015) broke down the emotion regulation process into its components and presented it in a multidimensional process model. According to Sheppes and colleagues (2015), emotions can be understood as internal changes that lead to external responses that have been shown to be beneficial from an evolutionary perspective. The multisystemic changes can be distinguished in terms of their intensity (strong–weak), duration (minutes, hours), frequency (frequency of occurrence in a given time), or type of reaction (quality of feeling).

The emotion regulation process can be roughly divided into an *emotion generation phase* (bottom-up) and an emotion *regulation phase* (top-down) (see Table 2). In the emergence phase, the emotional response is built up, and in the regulation phase, regulatory processes are activated to adapt the emotional response to the situation at hand and to the desired goal. In both phases, individual differences may represent vulnerability factors for the development of mental disorders (Gross, 2015; Sheppes et al., 2015).

Table 2. Emotion regulation phases according to Gross (2015)

Phases of emotion regulation	What happens during this phase?
Emotion build-up phase	1. Change in the world of the individual (world) 2. Perception of the change (perception) 3. Evaluation as positive or negative (validation) 4. Initiation of a reaction (action)
Emotion regulation phase	1. Identification phase: reaction required or not? 2. Selection phase: Which regulatory strategies are possible? 3. Implementation phase: strategy selection and implementation 4. Monitoring phase: continuous observation of the effects and adaptation of the strategy

Emotion Build-Up Phase

Emotional reactions are triggered by the perception of a threat in a person's world (internal or external). This is accompanied by experienced physiological or behavioral changes. According to the extended process model of emotion regulation (Gross, 2015), this process consists of four components (see Table 2): (1) a triggering aspect in the individual's world in the form of a change, (2) the perception of this change, (3) the evaluation as positive or negative, and (4) an initiated response.

Individual differences in the development of emotions are therefore already to be expected in the perception and evaluation of changes in the world and the rough classification into "good" or "bad." Existing negative schemas and unfavorable learned associations can strongly influence attentional, perceptual, and evaluative processes and increase the experience of threat in general, but also in specific situations, thereby initiating the strength of emotional reactions (Hofmann, 2019). Even in the context of expectancy-based approaches, according to which mental disorders are generally defined as disorders of expectations, individual differences lead to the formation of different expectations that negatively affect the further adjustment process (Rief, 2020). For example, someone with panic attacks will expect a catastrophe and act accordingly (e.g., call 911) rather than trusting that the anxiety will go away. Or a depressed person may not even try to change their situation due to a negative expectation of the future.

Emotion Regulation Phase

This primary process of emotion generation is followed by processes of emotion regulation (Gross, 2015). The emotion regulation phase can be divided into four phases (see Table 2). Each of these phases also includes a perception, evaluation, and reaction process.

The *identification phase* determines whether a reaction is required or not. Individual differences can arise here because, for example, alexithymic people do not perceive or recognize relevant signals from the environment and therefore underreact. On the other hand, people with a low tolerance for distress and high sensitivity are more likely to overreact. Also, strong fusion with existing negative schemas can distort the evaluation of situations. Learned helplessness may prevent information from this regulatory phase from being further processed (Hofmann, 2019; Sheppes et al., 2015).

The *selection phase* determines which strategies are available for emotion regulation. From a behavioral perspective, links to maladaptive regulatory mechanisms may be overrepresented (Dixon & Rehfeldt, 2018). For example, situations that produce negative affect may be associated with bulimic eating episodes or drug use through classical conditioning. Additionally, these may be operantly reinforced, e.g., through negative reinforcement mechanisms or incomplete feedback loops that only consider short-term consequences (Dixon & Rehfeldt, 2018; Sheppes et al., 2015). For example, a bulimic client may couple the reinforcing drop in tension following an eating episode with vomiting but may not make the connection between vomiting and other long-term negative consequences (e.g., social consequences, negative self-appraisal).

In the *implementation phase*, a decision is made as to which strategy is selected and applied. Again, individual differences in the perception or evaluation of strategies as a result of existing cognitive schemas may promote maladaptive use of strategies (De Houwer et al., 2018). In generalized anxiety disorder, the positive metacognition "thinking helps solve problems" leads to individuals sticking to this strategy during unpleasant emotional states, although the strategy becomes part of the problem, when recursive thinking turns into rumination (Wells, 2009). In a depressed state, the problem at this stage lies in the difficulty to access and activate positive emotional network regions as one possible strategy to distance oneself from a negative emotional state. This is a restriction found on a process level described by Hayes and colleagues (2015), where depressed individuals are not only entrapped in their negative network, but also shielded from positive network regions (see Figure 23 in Section 2.7.6). Finally, lack of knowledge of regulatory strategies has been blamed for the development of emotional problems (Papa et al., 2018; Sheppes et al., 2015). A limited repertoire reduces regulatory flexibility and is thus a significant vulnerability factor. As a consequence, treatment programs for "emotional skills training" (Berking & Whitley, 2014) have been developed for clinical practice so that affected individuals are specifically supported in this phase of the regulatory process.

In the *monitoring phase*, the effects of the regulation attempts are evaluated and adjusted. Limited competencies in this phase can lead to a failure to evaluate and adjust the use of strategies on an ongoing basis. The monitoring phase requires that operant factors be considered when adjusting strategies (Bonanno & Burton, 2013; Harvey et al., 2009). As a result of misjudgment, (1) effective strategies may be abandoned too early, (2) switching between effective strategies may occur too quickly, or (3) rigid adherence to an ineffective strategy may occur. Disruptions in these feedback processes have been identified in the development of chronic depression (McCullough, 2003). Referring to Piaget's developmental theory (Montada, 1995), McCullough (2003) postulated that chronically depressed individuals are cognitively at a preoperational stage and therefore direct their response predominantly ego-centered. That means that their reaction is formed solely from their own perspective, similar to how 5- to 9-year-olds react: "I hit him with a ruler because he called me stupid." This has an ego-centered logic. If someone hurts me, I hurt them back. Later on, people develop the ability to adjust their reaction by taking into account the consequences and directing their behavior towards desired goals. An older child might feel the desire to hurt the other person but they are able to understand that hitting someone leads to more conflict. At this higher cognitive level, the child may say: "If you continue to insult me, I will tell the teacher. But I'd prefer to be friends."

For the process-based approach, an ongoing, dynamic process is only possible through continuous feedback loops. This requires functioning cross-fading feedback loops at the cognitive, emotional, behavioral, physiological, and contextual levels. The result is a constant stream of monitored regulatory mechanisms. This dynamic character is captured in Gross' (2015) extended process model of emotion regulation.

Temperament

In developmental psychology, temperament is understood as a biology-related component of personality that is already observable in the first months of life and characterizes a person's typical experience and behavior across situations and across time (Petermann & Ulrich, 2019; Thomas & Chess, 1980).

Table 3 provides an overview of important individual differences in temperament (after Thomas & Chess, 1980) that are determinants of psychosocial adaptability. Thus, people have different starting points, and they have quite different coping options available to them.

Table 3. Dimensions of temperament according to Thomas and Chess (1980)

Temperament dimension	Expressions (endpoints of the dimension)
Activity level	high–low
Rhythm	regular–irregular
Distractibility	high–low
Initial reaction in new situations	approach–retreat
Adaptability	high–low
Perseverance and attention	long–short
Reaction intensity	high–low
Sensitivity	high–low
Mood quality	positive–negative

Of particular importance for emotional reactions are the predisposed mood quality, i.e., whether someone tends to have an enduring positive or negative affect, the degree of emotional sensitivity, and the intensity of the readiness to react. People with high sensitivity are hit with greater force by unpleasant situations than people with low sensitivity. Combined with a readiness to react intensely, it is more difficult to deal constructively with such a situation. If a person has several unfavorable temperamental characteristics, it is as if they were the only one competing in a race with tied shoelaces against professional runners with spikes.

Negative Affect

Negative affect has already been described as a vulnerability mechanism in the diathesis model further developed by Barlow and colleagues (2014). In this context, negative affect tends to be associated with avoidant tendencies and withdrawal (Hofmann, 2019). The unfavorable effect of avoidance behavior is discussed in more detail in Section 4.3 on response mechanisms. At this point, the effect of unbalanced affect shifted toward the negative pole is important because people with more positive affect orient more toward approach goals, whereas people with negative affect orient more toward avoidance goals. Positive affect is also associated with subjective well-being, which is associated with stronger bonds and attachment to social groups (Myers, 2000).

Under the influence of negative affect, the control of regulatory processes is markedly impaired, so that improvement of affect in therapy may be crucial for the implementation and maintenance of change.

Disregulation of Negative Affect: Rumination and Worry

Wells (2009) has described the importance of unproductive cognitive strategies in dealing with emotional problems and postulates this maladaptive metacognitive control as a vulnerability mechanism for the development and maintenance of numerous mental disorders. For example, the rigid positive metacognition, "If I just intensely and accurately analyze my problems and look for a solution, I will solve the problems" leads people to use these strategies for emotional problems, even when they are not effective. Rumination and worrying lead to the reinforcement of chronic negative affect states and to experiences of helplessness in the face of coping with the problems in focus (Rozanski & Kubzansky, 2005). The processes involved appear to be self-perpetuating: Rumination and worry promote negative affect and vice versa. They are relevant from a process-based perspective because, on the one hand, they promote negative affect and increase the risk of emotion regulation disorders through this activation of the negative affect system (Barlow, 2014). On the other hand, this inflexible use of an unproductive strategy initiates equally unproductive processing loops, like withdrawn behavior, that further build up multimodally across other system levels (Hayes, 2015).

Emotional Granularity

Emotional granularity (Suvak et al., 2011; Tugade et al., 2004) refers to the ability to differentially distinguish between emotional states. Is someone able to perceive and describe emotional states with a high degree of resolution, or do they only categorize as "good" and "bad"? Is the person able to notice fine gradations in the intensity of feelings? This can help to endure an unpleasant situation when one notices that the intensity of an emotion is slowly decreasing. Emotional granularity can be captured well with an intensity-valence matrix (see Figure 30). While some people have a differentiated emotional life at their disposal, others operate with crude "good–bad" and "strong–weak" categories. Although there is only limited research on this concept, we believe it is very useful for understanding and treating emotional disorders. As explained in Section 4.2.7 on the regulatory flexibility model, the possible fine gradations in perception and response are critical to the ability to fine-tune one's own responses as well (Bonanno & Burton, 2013).

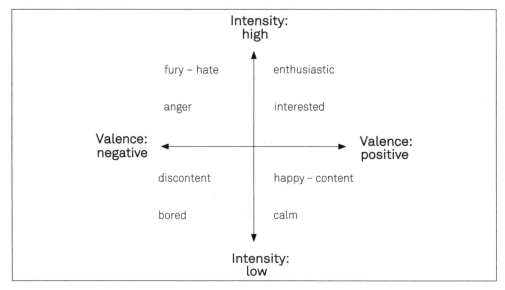

Figure 30. Valence–intensity matrix of emotion perception and naming.

Alexithymia

The alexithymia concept refers to the difficulty in perceiving and describing emotions and in distinguishing between feelings and physical sensations. In further development of this concept (Taylor & Bagby, 2000), it was defined more generally as a deficit in the cognitive processing and regulation of emotions. When asked, "What feelings did the criticism from your supervisor elicit in you?" an alexithymic client looked helpless and replied, "Hmm? I was tired and left." Alexithymic individuals are also less able to perceive and categorize interpersonal tensions and are unable to communicate them verbally or mimically (Taylor & Bagby, 2000). Thus, this vulnerability factor also operates at the interpersonal level.

Alexithymic people have little or only very blurred emotional information available to them when coping with demands and stressors. Therefore, they also find it difficult to name emotional problems, to ask for help or to recognize the added value of therapy. As a result, they have difficulty distinguishing between adaptive and less adaptive emotion regulation strategies. In difficult emotional situations, they therefore do not try to get to the bottom of feelings or talk to someone.

From a process-oriented perspective, alexithymic individuals lack crucial emotional information for shaping and regulating processual responses to difficult situations. They have low emotional granularity and poor perception of emotional feedback loops, and their repertoire of responses is also less finely tuned, so that the flexible regulation of demands is significantly impaired (Bonanno & Burton, 2013).

Emotional Clarity

Emotional clarity is, in a sense, the opposite of alexithymia. It refers to awareness and understanding of one's emotions and the ability to name them (Gohm & Clore, 2000).

A lack of emotional clarity can be caused not only by "too little" feeling, but also by "too much" feeling, as in emotionally unstable personality disorder. Emotional experience is complex and dynamic and can be very confusing for the sufferer. In PTSD treatment resulting from intrafamilial sexual abuse, it is often very difficult for victims to clearly name the multitude of conflicting feelings related to the perpetrator: Fear, disgust, closeness, love, anger, shame, arousal, and guilt overlap to form a blurry emotional knot. Obtaining clarity about the simultaneity of conflicting emotional states is a therapy-enhancing process in this context (Kircanski et al., 2012).

Emotional Intelligence

Emotional intelligence combines the above-mentioned skills. It includes the abilities to (1) assess and express emotions, (2) regulate emotions, and (3) use emotions in solving problems (Mayer & Salovey, 1997). While emotional granularity and empathy are essential for the first factor, using emotions to solve problems requires additional creativity and flexibility in thinking, as well as the ability to direct attention and motivation to target states (Mayer & Salovey, 1997). Thus, the concept of emotional intelligence combines individual prerequisites in terms of the differentiated perception of feelings and the necessary cognitive, social, and communicative abilities to use emotions adaptively in coping with demands.

Reduced Stress Tolerance

Reduced stress tolerance is reflected in a reduced tolerance for enduring unpleasant internal states, such as unpleasant or intense feelings or sensations. Stress tolerance is a key skill for understanding feelings. It allows one to experience unpleasant states without becoming overwhelmed by them and unable to act (Hofmann, 2019). Especially in the case of difficult and sometimes overwhelming demands, the person thus gains time and can postpone impulsive reactions in order to gain clarity about the event and fine-tune the response. Limiting the stress response increases the likelihood for experiential avoidance (McHugh et al., 2013). Reduced stress tolerance can relate to unpleasant thoughts, physical states, or feelings, with intolerance for negative feelings playing a central role in the development of numerous disorders (Frank & Davidson, 2014). As a vulnerability mechanism, these limitations lead to the maintenance of anxiety disorders (Keough et al., 2010), addictions (Richards et al., 2011), and eating disorders (Anestis et al., 2012), and they activate maladaptive response processes, such as withdrawal behavior, rumination, and emotion suppression or emotion-avoidant processes (see Frank & Davidson, 2014).

Low Uncertainty Tolerance

Low stress tolerance for *uncertainty* is a well-documented vulnerability mechanism for the development of anxiety disorders and depression (see Frank & Davidson, 2014). Uncertainty intolerance is defined as the tendency to react negatively emotionally, cognitively, and behaviorally to ambiguous situations (Dugas et al., 2004). In line with the constructs mentioned so far, this mechanism leads to new situations being interpreted more

68   Chapter 4

as threats and experienced as less predictable. It therefore promotes worry processes, a negative focus on problems, and cognitive avoidance (Buhr & Dugas, 2012).

High Anxiety Sensitivity

Low tolerance for *anxiety*, or heightened anxiety sensitivity, represents one of the three central fears in Reiss and McNally's fear-expectancy model (after Reiss, 1991). It refers to the fear of anxiety due to the belief that fears will lead to inevitable negative physical, cognitive, or social consequences. In addition to this fear of anxiety, fear of injury or illness and fear of evaluation are critical in shaping anxiety in the fear-expectancy model. High *anxiety sensitivity* can be evaluated as a well-documented transdiagnostic vulnerability mechanism (Frank & Davidson, 2014); it increases the likelihood of panic disorder, general anxiety, phobias, and substance abuse (Reiss, 1991) and may predict depressive symptoms. Thus, decreasing anxiety sensitivity is an overarching therapeutic goal for many disorders (see Frank & Davidson, 2014).

Low stress tolerance for *evaluations* promotes the development of emotional problems associated with shame, guilt, worry (Frank & Davidson, 2014), and fear of rejection (Gilbert, 2005). Fear of being negatively evaluated is a documented vulnerability mechanism for social anxiety (Clark & Wells, 1995), eating disorders (Utschig et al., 2010), and PTSD (Collimore et al., 2009), among others.

Affective Styles

Affective styles are a type of response schema and describe the ways in which people cope with emotional demands. For Davidson and Begley (2012), people differ in terms of their affective styles on six subdimensions. These relate to different abilities (e.g., the ability to decode and interpret nonverbal cues) that vary in strength among people. Table 4 summarizes the six subdimensions. A person's affective style results from the combination of individually expressed abilities of all subdimensions. For example, someone may be slow to recover from emotional shocks but have a more positive perception of the world.

Table 4. Affective styles according to Davidson and Begley (2012)

Subdimensions of affective styles	Description
Resilience	Determines how quickly or slowly someone recovers from an emotional upset
Outlook	Refers to the tendency to perceive the world as more positive or more negative
Social intuition	Ability to decode and interpret nonverbal signals
Self-awareness	Accuracy with which internal physical signals are decoded
Sensitivity to context	Ability to adapt emotional reactions to the context
Attention	Ability to keep attention focused and not get distracted

As a result of the predisposed affective style, people have very different prerequisites for responding to emotional demands. The affective styles listed in Table 4 determine the basis for the regulatory flexibility described in Section 4.2.7 (Bonanno & Burton, 2013).

Emotional Flexibility

Emotional flexibility refers to the ability to adapt one´s emotion regulation to the challenging situation (Hofmann, 2019). Psychological flexibility in general represents a core dimension when it comes to understanding coping processes. It is not that one particular strategy or response is superior to another across situations but rather that it is important to flexibly adjust one's response on an ongoing basis depending on the outcome. Cheng (2001) examined flexibility in coping with emotionally distressing stressors under controlled experimental conditions. He found considerable variability in identifying stressors, assessing the controllability of stressors, and variability in selecting strategies. Emotional flexibility is also associated with better adaptive performance and less anxiety and depression (Cheng, 2003).

4.2.3   Behavioral Level

Learning processes form the DNA of both cognitive behavioral therapy (CBT) and process-based therapy. Mental disorders are unfavorable network linkages that develop and are maintained through associative learning and operant reinforcement mechanisms. Learning processes shape visible behavior, as well as cognitive, emotional, physiological, and interpersonal network linkages (Dixon & Rehfeldt, 2018).

Barlow's vulnerability model (Suárez et al., 2009) for the development of emotional disorders views earlier learning processes as predisposing to the development of mental disorders. In addition to the biological factors already mentioned, early learning experiences in which stressful life events were experienced as unpredictable and uncontrollable lead to the formation of generalized schemas according to which new demands are generally evaluated as unpredictable and uncontrollable and thus as potentially threatening. These schemata represent a risk factor for coping with future demands. A predisposition for anxiety disorders developed in this way can explain why someone develops an anxiety disorder later in life – but not how it is individually shaped. Depending on individual contextual factors, anxiety may relate to social situations, result in body-related health fears, or lead to panic attacks in confined spaces.

Classical Conditioning: Stimulus–Response Linkages

Classical conditioning, i.e., the establishment of links through the temporal association of stimuli, explains why previously unconditioned stimuli become conditioned stimuli. In this way, favorable – but also unfavorable – S-R links are learned effortlessly. Our brains are constantly busy linking things that occur together so that a network of associations emerges from them (Bennett & Oliver, 2019; Dixon & Rehfeldt, 2018; Frank & Davidson, 2014).

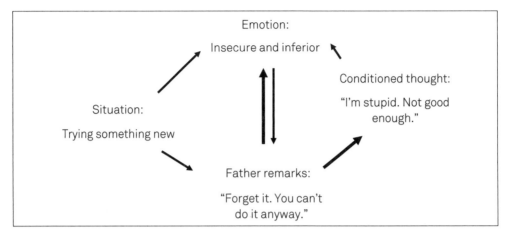

Figure 31. Simple associative network through classical conditioning that constitutes a stable network over time.

A pathological network consists of many such multimodal unfavorable S-R connections. The more often associations are repeated, the stronger the S-R connections of the network. In this way, ruminative processes or avoidance behaviors cause people to mentally repeat and generalize existing negative associations. The more unfavorable S-R connections a pathological network has, the more difficult it will be to change that network. Figure 31 shows a simple network formed by a classically conditioned linkage between a new situation, a feeling of insecurity, and a negative self-evaluation. Such a linkage can become more and more consolidated through repetition, generalization, and relational learning. If a child hears the phrase, "Don't do that, you can't do it anyway," when trying something new, and wonders if it might be stupid, then this thought will be activated every time the child tries something new. Since children are always trying something new as they develop, this thought becomes associated with many situations and feelings of insecurity, hindering the development of helpful networks.

In this way, habits are established that control our behavior automatically and subconsciously. These habits help us as long as everything goes according to plan. If the situation requires a change in our behavioral responses, habits hinder flexible alignment with a desired goal (Wood, 2019).

Individual differences in establishing or loosening associations may have unfavorable effects on association learning and thus constitute vulnerability mechanisms (see Box 1).

Box 1. Individual differences in classical conditioning that may represent vulnerability mechanisms

> a) *Unfavorable S-R linkages are rigid and resistant to change:* The affected person is attached to these established linkages. This is the case, among other things, with personality disorders in which enduring patterns of perceiving and reacting to demands are rigid and override what is currently experienced.
> b) *Newly learned adaptive associations and links are unstable:* As a result, the person is distractible and cannot deepen the new learned associations. This often occurs in therapy, when clients pick up new ideas and are able to show changes in a therapy session, but in the next session cannot recall what they were able to grasp a week earlier. The new associations allowing changes remained superficial or unstable.

c) *Low flexibility in establishing and disconnecting S-R linkages:* Adaptive responses often require flexible, differential connecting and loosening of existing linkages. This includes the ability to maintain single, functional links in a network while at the same time loosening unfavorable links. The more finely I can separate individual connections in the network and create new connections with a better fit, the more customized the result.

d) *Overgeneralization of S-R links neglecting feedback loops:* Too rapid generalization of learned associations to new situations can be problematic, especially if context information of the new situation and reality-related feedback does not tailor the response pattern. This is the case, for example, when a traumatization results in the overgeneralized belief that it is important to never again trust another person, neglecting the fact that people can represent both a threat and an important source of protection, safety, and comfort. The lack of discriminative learning poses a limitation for overcoming trauma.

Operant Conditioning: Feedback Loops

Reinforcement processes (or operant conditioning processes) are relevant for the establishment and consolidation of new connections and are significant as a mechanism for the maintenance of behavior. Essential to this is operant feedback. This requires that feedback processes function between system levels and that the information can be used to modify behavior (Frank & Davidson, 2014). Access to these feedback loops can be impeded by alexithymia or low emotional clarity. In a way, without feedback loops, learning is almost impossible. If you practice playing darts, but you are blindfolded and do not get the feedback where your dart landed, you can practice as much as you want, you do not have the information you need to improve. For these people life is like flying a plane without the necessary instruments indicating the flight altitude, velocity, or take-off speed. This reduced ability to use information from feedback loops to model adaptive responses represents a vulnerability factor that impairs learning, adaptation, and regulatory flexibility (Bonanno & Burton, 2013).

Susceptibility to negative reinforcement. Behavior is primarily reinforced or extinguished by positive and negative consequences. Of particular importance is the absence of feared negative consequences as reinforcers because this establishes avoidance behavior. Initially, avoidance behavior prevents contact with the environment, which in turn causes this avoidance behavior to continue – even when the triggering reason no longer exists (Dixon & Rehfeldt, 2018; Frank & Davidson, 2014). Again, the detrimental effect on ongoing learning from the lack of reality-based feedback loops focused on long-term consequences is essential to the disruption of regulatory flexibility (Bonanno & Burton, 2013).

Level of cognitive development. The ability to direct one's own behavior toward long-term desired consequences requires numerous subfunctions, such as frustration tolerance, executive functions, and also the ability to maintain an internal representation of the desired target state. At the same time, different effects at different system levels must be accounted for with different time courses. Thus, a reaction may trigger aversive feelings and be associated with interpersonal conflict in the short term but have positive effects on the same relationship and enhance one's sense of self-efficacy in the medium- to long-term perspective. Keeping track of and accounting for the numerous interacting consequences is a complex undertaking (Dixon & Rehfeldt, 2018; Harvey et al., 2009). Piaget's cognitive stages of cognitive development (Montada, 1995) classify individuals who orient their behavior predominantly toward immediate consequences at a preoperational level. On this level, an individual cannot sufficiently anticipate operant feedback information to constantly develop more refined reactions, but is confined to once learned responses, even if they are maladaptive to the situation. Asking a client why he hit his neighbor although on parole, he replied, "Because he insulted my family." The consequence of eventually going back to jail is not accessible, so responding to an insult by fighting back feels as the only right thing to do. Not sufficiently developed operant learning skills result in problem-solving attempts falling short, staying immature, or contributing to interpersonal problems. The impairment of operant feedback learning has shown to be a core vulnerability process responsible for the development of chronic depression. Helping sufferers to cope with their operant learning disorder and to direct their behavior toward desired long-term consequences is a core process in cognitive behavioral analysis system of psychotherapy (CBASP) treatment of chronic depression (McCullough, 2003).

Social Learning and Model Learning

A parallel process to the classical and operant learning mechanisms mentioned earlier are processes of social learning or model learning, which occurs through observing and imitating others. In clinical practice, this is relevant as a vulnerability factor, as therapeutic reinforcers are not infrequently at odds with clients' social reinforcers (Bennett & Oliver, 2019; Dixon & Rehfeldt, 2018; Frank & Davidson, 2014;).

Within an addiction treatment setting, addiction- and offense-free living may be reinforced. This may be of little use if outside the therapy setting these self-harming behaviors are reinforced through social learning and model learning. For example, a client with addiction problems experiences in their circle of friends that the feeling of belongingness as an important social reinforcer is linked to shared drug use or to acquisitive crime. Or, children with aggression problems experience in their peer group that status and recognition come through the exercise of violence, while de-escalation strategies learned in therapy result in ridicule in their social environment.

There are many such examples where a pathological behavior represents an adaptation to a pathological system and therefore change within that system is difficult to maintain against the flow of social learning processes. Social learning processes may thus represent a core process that maintains disorders (Hofmann & Hayes, 2018). Measures to effect change may include distancing oneself from the previous circle of friends or creating an environment conducive to learning (e.g., therapeutic residential community).

4.2.4 Cognitive Level

With the recognition of the cognitive dimension in psychopathology and psychotherapy a wealth of research emerged on cognitive processes that may condition mental health problems. Unfavorable attributional patterns, negative thinking, dichotomous thinking, catastrophizing, personalizing, and other thinking disorders have been identified as important vulnerability factors in the development and maintenance of mental disorders (see Barlow, 2014). Self-generated expectations, anticipated consequences, or latent and implicit cognitive processes create cognitive traces and form cognitive schemas that influence emotional states and behaviors (see Beck, 1967; Ellis, 1989). Through symbolic learning, rules and relations can expand cognitive representations to new situations without subjecting them to a reality test. Thus, disconnecting the learning process from experience and shifting learning completely on a symbolic level. Symbolic learning enables a quantum leap for experience-independent learning in favorable cases but can lead to the propagation of unfavorable relations if important cognitive subfunctions are in some way impaired (De Houwer et al., 2018).

Memory Processes

Systematic differences in the storage and use of memory content are effective vulnerability factors on a transdiagnostic level. A bias in selective storage of unfavorable memory content, overgeneralization of disorder-relevant memory content, and cognitive avoidance in retrieval and decoding of disorder-relevant information promote the development of disorders (Harvey et al., 2009). When suffering from a mental disorder like depression or anxiety, affected individuals tend to remember more negative aspects and are less able to access alternative, helpful information.

From the network perspective, network structures relevant to the disorder are activated and/or positive memory areas of the network are inhibited. Since memory content and processes are the basis for learning processes, the formation of expectations, and cognitive schemas, distortions in the area of memory can lead to distortions at other process levels and contribute to the development of psychopathology (Harvey et al., 2009).

Cognitive Fusion Tendency

In a cognitive fused state, we confuse our thoughts with reality and forget that they are "only" thoughts. We "clump" or "merge" with our thinking. We do not experience ourselves thinking, but it is as if we are the thought. For affected people there is no difference between having the thought of passing out and passing out in reality. If we confuse our thinking with reality, our thoughts override our perception of reality. This insulates us from corrective experiences (see Bennett & Oliver, 2019). Wells (2009) has described the effects of fusion or defusion (detached mindfulness) for the development of depression and anxiety, and in the ACT approach (Hayes et al., 2009), fusion represents one of six core disorder-maintaining processes in the Hexaflex model.

Essential from a process-based perspective is that cognitive fusion (1) makes thinking inflexible, (2) fosters processing that is distant from reality, which (3) makes one resistant to change through fusion with content. For example, if one is highly fused with the thought of "being worthless," this easily creates a pull that narrows one's view of oneself and the world to this premise: Not only is the proposition thought but the annihilating dimension of the thought is felt (Wells, 2009).

Thus, the cognitive vulnerability factors described in the following sections are most significant if the person is also fused with the cognitive patterns or content.

Negative Schemes

Cognitive schemas are defined following Piaget (see Montada, 1995) as relatively stable, conscious or unconscious basic assumptions that control information processing and behavior. They are goal- and action-oriented, accompanied by emotions, and lead to characteristic cognitions. Rigid schemas increase the propensity to develop mental disorders. Thus, dysfunctional schemas lead to false basic assumptions regarding relevant areas of self and life and thus to inadequate patterns of processing and behavior.

Negative schemas, as described by Beck's depression model (1967), are negative internal representations of oneself ("I am worthless"), others ("I cannot trust others"), the world ("The world is threatening and punishing"), and the future ("Things will not get better"). They are activated by external events or emotional states. Thus, these schemas determine the threat content of normal events and the formation of expectations. Both are crucial for the development of mental disorders (Rief, 2020). Failure may for example activate a negative self-schema and causes this event to become a threat to the self. At the same time, it confirms the expectation that one is not good enough, the future is negative, and other people are judgmental and not to be trusted (Dixon & Rehfeldt, 2018).

Extent of Negative Thinking

Kendall and colleagues (1989) have examined the power of "non-negative thinking" as a safeguard against psychopathology. They emphasize the harmfulness of negative, self-referential thoughts. Following their State-of-Mind (SOM) model, they calculated a co-efficient relating positive and negative self-referential thoughts. In the most adaptive cognitive state, this coefficient is 0.62, meaning that positive self-references are at least 62%. In this state, the individual is in "successful coping dialogue" (Schwartz, 1997). Schwartz revised the SOM model; according to his model, the optimal range is 85–90% positive self-statements. The SOM model points to the particular importance of negative thinking as a vulnerability factor in the development of psychopathology.

The role of *dysfunctional attributional processes* as a vulnerability factor is well established across disorders (Beck, 1967). Studies show a negative bias in the perception of disorder-relevant stimuli such that more negative expectations and fewer positive expectations are generated. As a result, feared associations are overestimated (Harvey et al., 2009). Frank and Davidson (2014) also identify systematic inflexible attribution biases as relevant to disorders, which can be both internal ("It's all my fault") and inflexible external ("It's not my fault. Others are to blame").

If attribution processes are systematically distorted, similar errors in activating coping responses will occur again and again. If causes of problems are attributed unchecked to internal, stable characteristics of my person over which I have little influence, and at the same time I assess the consequences as exaggeratedly negative, then it will be difficult to activate motivational processes that help me to actively cope with the problem.

Negative control beliefs about unpleasant events and sensations as an enduring schema resulting from formative negative experiences represent a vulnerability mechanism for emotional disorders. The negative schema leads to the interpretation of new demands and events as not controllable (Chorpita & Barlow, 1998), thus influencing the choice of response mechanisms. If I do not believe I can influence something, I am more likely to respond with avoidance, escape, or emotion suppression than if I have high control beliefs.

This results in a *negative problem orientation*. These are stable, generalized cognitive-emotional reaction patterns to problems. People with a negative problem orientation are more likely to perceive problems as a threat and are more likely to evaluate problems as unsolvable. They doubt that they can contribute to the solution themselves and are more quickly frustrated by problems. This reduces self-efficacy expectations and motivation to actively tackle problems with the expected negative consequences for the coping process (see Frank & Davidson, 2014).

For example, an exaggerated belief that things are one's responsibility and an exaggerated appraisal of the potential for threat represents a well-documented vulnerability factor for numerous anxiety and obsessive-compulsive disorders (Salkovskis et al., 1999), as well as for depression and worry.

Metacognitive Processes and Beliefs

There are a number of generally very harmful and stressful thought processes that lead to fusion with unfavorable thoughts, promote regulatory inflexibility, amplify the effect of unfavorable thought content, and are insulated from reality-based feedback mechanisms. Well-documented maladaptive metacognitive functioning includes recursive thinking in the sense of worrying as a process, rumination, and "postevent processing," and, furthermore, cognitive avoidance through thought control, thought suppression, and worrying as a function (Frank & Davidson, 2014). These thought processes are unproductive and result in negative cycles that cause intended problem-solving attempts to contribute to the reinforcement of these problems. Fighting worry with worry leads to further increases in worry. If one tries to ban worry thoughts in response, this strategy also results in an intensified worry cycle. Such cognitive processes are controlled at a metacognitive level (Wells, 2009) by positive and negative metacognitions. Positive metacognitions are beliefs about the positive effects of thinking, such as, "If I just think enough, I'll find a solution." This belief is the metacognitive basis of rumination and rumination processes (Wells, 2009). Negative metacognitions are beliefs about the negative impact of thinking processes, such as worrying about going crazy if one fails to stop thinking. This usually triggers cognitive control, suppression, or avoidance responses, all of which lead to reinforcement of toxic cognitive activity (Harvey et al., 2009; Wells, 2009).

Symbolic Learning Processes: Learning and Language

Much research has examined the role of language in learning processes and has shown that the learning processes outlined earlier are independent of experience and can be shifted to a cognitive level through symbolic processes of thought and language (Hayes et al., 2001). Studies were able to show that verbal prompts overrode the effect of actual reinforcer contingencies. In a nutshell, symbolic processes allow for decoupling from real reinforcer processes and allow for new linkages to emerge through abstract establishment of relations.

The relational frame theory (Hayes, 2004), which derived from these theories on symbolic learning, explains how behavior can explain the development of psychological or somatic responses through symbolic linkage at the linguistic level alone. In a study by Dougher and colleagues (2007), one experimental group learned that $X<Y<Z$, and the

other that X, Y, Z were unrelated. Both groups were then shocked by aversive stimuli in the presence of "Y" and showed a physiological fear response. "X" elicited no particular response in either group, whereas the group participants who had learned that "Y" was smaller than "Z" developed a stronger physiological response to "Z" – without ever having had any negative experience with it. They generalized the relation on a symbolic level to other system levels (physiological).

Especially from a network perspective, these findings are interesting, because once a problematic pattern is established, this pattern can spread unhindered through this symbolic level, contributing to the elaboration of a pathological network on other system levels – like a computer virus that has invaded the operating system and rewrites the programs – including the history.

4.2.5 Level of the Self

The regulatory processes described so far at the cognitive, emotional, and behavioral levels are closely linked to self-related processes. The concept of the self goes back to William James (1890/1983), who divides the "I" into both an object (which is recognized) and a subject (which recognizes). The object is called "self," the cognizing subject "I." The "I" can experience the self, observe and evaluate internal states, and experience itself as an agent of its own actions. The self-concept presupposes that the person distinguishes between himself and the environment, that other people also have a self, and that it is possible to take the respective perspectives.

According to the ACT approach (Bennett & Oliver, 2019; Hayes et al., 2009), the self consists of three dimensions:
(1) The "self as content" describes the content dimensions of all internal experiences, such as thoughts, memories, and perceptions.
(2) The "self as context" is the space in which this content takes place.
(3) The "self as process" describes the process dimension, i.e., the way in which the content and the context are viewed.

Inflexibility of the Self (Including Personality Disorders)

As a metaphor for this dimension, one can imagine a room (context), in which there is furniture (content), and which one can illuminate with a flashlight (process). Problematic in a psychopathological sense is when we forget that we are more than the content of our inner processes and the thoughts about us (e.g., "I am shy") and this dominates our self-perception and behavior. A fusion with our self-image occurs, and we do not realize that our representation of our self is just a story of us, alongside which many others can exist. This distinction is important because otherwise our cognitive representation of our self narrows our regulatory flexibility and repertoire of response options (Bennett & Oliver, 2019; Hayes et al., 2009).

For people who work in helping professions and are strongly fused with their professionally shaped self-image, problems can arise in this way: "I don't need any help! I am the one who has to be strong. I help others in need and must not have any weaknesses" are statements that show how strongly the content of the "story about oneself" constricts

Core Processes of Psychopathology 77

the person concerned. Adaptive in the sense of the process-based approach is a flexible and distanced relationship to one's content self. For example, an affected person might then recognize, "In my role as a firefighter, I'm often the helper and show strength, and *I* need help with things that require softer skills rather than strength."

Negative Self-Focused Attention

According to Pyszczynski and Greenberg (1987) negative self-focused attention can be viewed as a core process leading to an individual experiencing depressive symptoms. The latter occurs when a person gets stuck in a self-regulatory adaptation process and fails to reduce the discrepancy to a desired goal state. In the sense the self is a spectator of its own failure to cope with a situation, leading to feelings of helplessness and sadness. According to this theory, continuous self-awareness of a failing regulatory attempt is responsible for negative affect and self-esteem loss. Recent theories specify that private self-focus is more associated with depression (sadness, helplessness), whereas public self-focus is more associated with social anxiety (Mor & Winquist, 2002).

In this concept, the self takes on the monitoring function of regulatory processes, like a mental drone hovering over us evaluating the progress of our attempts to cope with demands. With the help of the self-focus, information about the current state, the desired target state, norm values, reactions of the environment and measures are collected and evaluated. The self determines when the self-regulatory process can be terminated or whether it must go through further loops. The positive or negative affect experienced depends on the outcome of the regulatory process. According to this, self-esteem says something about the evaluation of one's own regulatory apparatus. It is not for nothing that self-esteem is a central issue for the vast majority of clients in psychotherapy (Potreck-Rose, 2006). The self observes the failure of coping efforts. This generates dissatisfaction with self and partly explains feelings of guilt and shame, negative affect, or fears of being judged or rejected. In a way, our self watches us play the game of life and gets fed up and depressed when we appear to be losing the game.

4.2.6 Attachment and Relationship Level

Attachment theory postulates a genetically inherent need for attachment or closeness. Through early attachment experiences, an internal representation of the world and the relationship to the world is developed, which acts as a blueprint and shapes patterns of response in later relationships (Grossmann & Grossmann, 2004; Strauss, 2008).

This blueprint forms an inner working model. It includes expectations of others and evaluations of oneself. This primary filter of experience thus determines the potential threat content of the world and includes a basic schema regarding the relationship between me as an individual and the world (others). This filter explains individual differences regarding: How safe is the world? How much can I trust others? Will I be comforted or left alone when things are not going well for me? A secure attachment relationship leads to experiencing the world as a safe place, a place to explore on a foundation of emotional security. An insecure and especially a disorganized attachment does not provide this secure foundation. The mechanisms of information and affect processing first and foremost serve to protect against attachment-related pain (Grossmann & Grossmann, 2004).

Extensive studies show that secure attachment is associated with numerous benefits for self-regulatory adjustment processes, including increased emotion regulation capacity, a larger repertoire of coping and social skills, more openness, advantages in exploratory learning, better handling of unpleasant emotional states, and higher tolerance for errors and frustration. People with secure attachment focus problems better, are more cooperative, develop more positive working relationships, and show more sophisticated object perception. In contrast, insecure and disorganized attachment patterns exhibit defensive response mechanisms that affect all system levels and disrupt functional regulation (Grossmann & Grossmann, 2004). This leads to more hostility, less trust, and trivialization tendencies when the attachment structure is insecure, and to greater disruptions in life coping when the attachment representation is disorganized (Strauss, 2008). Attachment representation has been shown to influence the development of eating disorders (Soares et al., 2008), depression, somatoform disorders, and personality disorders (Grossmann & Grossmann, 2004).

4.2.7 Specific Constructs

Regulatory Flexibility

Although regulation processes can be viewed as dynamic, coping and regulation strategies are often divided into "good" and "bad" strategies. However, in a large meta-analysis of 306 studies (Webb et al., 2012), only weak differences on the level of strategies were shown with regard to emotion regulation. Thus, it is not the use of *specific* strategies that is crucial for successful emotion regulation, but the *flexible* use of strategies.

Bonanno and Burton (2013) emphasize the importance of individual differences in regulatory flexibility in their three-component model. Regulatory flexibility is understood here as an ongoing, multidimensional response process and may represent a vulnerability mechanism. Individual differences in regulatory flexibility can be explained by differences in context sensitivity, repertoire of strategies, and utility of feedback information. *Context sensitivity* refers to the ability to perceive demands and opportunities of the situation and adapt responses to ongoing contextual demands-rather than reacting normatively to individual triggers. The *repertoire component* includes the range of possible strategies available for responding to changing contextual demands. The *feedback component* includes the ability to attend to and evaluate the effects reported back in feedback loops and adjust strategy deployment accordingly. The three-component model is shown in Figure 32.

In the context of the process-based approach, this overarching concept is helpful for understanding the vulnerability processes presented so far. In principle, it is always a question of how flexible and adapted an individual can respond to environmental demands. Can it take into account the divergent effects on individual subsystems and activate responses that have long-term beneficial effects? Essential to this is a regulatory process that is able to continuously perceive, evaluate, and flexibly adapt various system information when planning and deploying strategies (Bonanno & Burton, 2013).

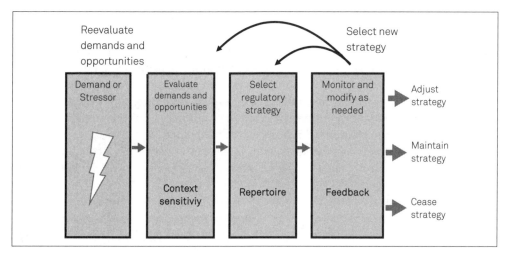

Figure 32. Three-component model of regulatory flexibility. Reprinted with permission from Bonanno and Burton, 2013, p. 595.

Perfectionism

Perfectionism is also a transdiagnostic vulnerability mechanism and is well documented for the maintenance and development of anxiety, depression, and eating disorders (Egan et al., 2011). It represents the counter-process to regulatory flexibility. Perfectionism in its clinical meaning describes the rigid pursuit of specific, self-imposed goals or standards in one or more areas of life and the dependence on their achievement. Such behavior may result in individuals being unable to adapt their goal setting and use of strategies to the context, i.e., not using information from multidimensional feedback loops for the regulatory process. This unproductive way of coping with demands leads at times to rigidly applying the same ineffective strategy. This naturally results in excesses or repeated failures, self-deprecation, and feelings of failure. Changing this perfectionistic coping pattern is therefore a central therapeutic goal in eating disorder, anxiety, and depression treatment (Egan et al., 2011).

4.3 Response Mechanisms

Response mechanisms are processes that are set in motion when demands meet vulnerability mechanisms and feedback loops continue to register a discrepancy between the current state and target state. In people with good regulatory flexibility, this is a background process. Such individuals are able to fine-tune their responses at each feedback loop, increasing their repertoire of strategies and their context sensitivity (Bonanno & Burton, 2013).

The following sections describe the most common responses that are transdiagnostically associated with the development psychopathology. They are not maladaptive per se, but they can set in motion unregulated vicious circles, unfavorable response cascades,

80   Chapter 4

or maladaptive inhibitory control processes, thus disrupting adaptive regulatory processes. Essentially, these are multidimensional avoidance responses that postpone unfavorable mental states in the short term but inevitably reinforce them in the long term.

The boundary between vulnerability and response mechanisms is sometimes blurred. Cognitive fusion as a vulnerability mechanism favors a pathological reaction. At the same time, fusion can be a reaction mechanism, for example, when someone tries to control an unsettling situation by a cognitive fusing rumination process. Table 5 provides an overview of the response mechanisms described in the following sections; we have attempted to divide them roughly by system level, with many of the responses involving multidimensional processes.

Table 5. Reaction mechanisms (core processes) at different system levels

System level	Reaction mechanisms (core processes)
Behavioral level	• Avoidance and escape behavior • Safety and reinsurance behavior • Obsessive-compulsive behavior • Overriding concept of experiential avoidance
Cognitive level	• Selective attention focus • Harmful thought processes and processes of metacognitive control • Cognitive avoidance through thought control and thought suppression • Cognitive avoidance through rumination, brooding and worrying • Cognitive fusion • Cognitive distorsions • Cognitive misattributions
Emotional level	• Emotional avoidance • Dysfunctional emotion regulation strategies
Motivational level	• State orientation (instead of approach motivation) • Avoidance motivation • Lack of connection with own value orientation
Social level and interaction level	• Interactions between interpersonal factors and individual psychopathology • Interpersonal regulation processes

4.3.1 Behavioral Core Processes

As described earlier, the fundamental behavioral mechanisms of behavior therapy (responsive and operant learning) are central in the context of process-based approaches. They explain at which point and under which conditions links in a complex network are established, maintained, tightened, and loosened and why these links are not unlearned even when they create suffering. They also explain how people can extend formative experiences to other areas of their lives by establishing relations (Dixon & Rehfeldt, 2018; Frank & Davidson, 2014). This section focuses on core behavioral processes that are initiated in response to the interaction of demand and vulnerability mechanisms.

Avoidance and Escape Behavior

Avoidance behavior, as a behavioral dimension of the concept of experiential avoidance (Hayes et al., 1996), is involved in the development and maintenance of mental disorders in a way that is overtly disturbing. The avoidance response is based on assumptions or evaluations about consequences of the feared situation (Beck, 1967) and aims to avoid unpleasant emotional states in the short term. In the case of anxiety, this may be the belief that one will die or lose control in certain situations, embarrass oneself by having a panic attack, or be unable to endure the anticipated anxiety or physical symptoms (Frank & Davidson, 2014).

Generally avoiding feared situations or the feeling of anxiety and escaping from these situations are problematic from a learning perspective because they prevent new learning experiences and prevent the correction of negative beliefs and experiences. Avoidance behavior is detrimental to adaptive regulation because, as a reflexive "all-or-nothing" response, it is not very context sensitive or flexible and is not regulated by feedback loops (Bonanno et al., 2004). It shifts the focus to internal experience and thus fosters other problematic processes such as recursive thinking and high self-attention. In the long term, avoidance is related to neglecting important life tasks and positive and social activities, social withdrawal, and the narrowing of perception to avoidance goals (Dixon & Rehfeldt, 2018; Harvey et al., 2009). Inactivity and withdrawal as a result of avoidance behaviors in depressive states also promote other negative effects, such as isolation, which in turn is associated with prompting further negative processes. As described earlier, disengagement from real-world conditions promotes generalization of unfavorable associations through symbolic learning processes (De Houwer et al., 2018; Dixon & Rehfeldt, 2018). In the case of anxiety, avoidance behavior undercuts the habituation process and thus a self-regulatory adaptive response as well as a build-up of anxiety-reducing control beliefs (see Harvey et al., 2009).

Safety and Reinsurance Behavior

Safety behaviors are behaviors that are used in situations to prevent fears or negative consequences that would otherwise occur. Corresponding behaviors are responsible for the fact that an anxiety network does not dissolve, although the feared consequences, such as fainting, never occur. In the affected client's logic, they would have fainted a thousand times over had they refrained from the safety behavior (Clark, 1999; Harvey et al., 2009).

Obsessive-Compulsive Behavior

Sometimes this avoidance behavior is masked by repetitive behaviors or thought processes that serve to mitigate unpleasant emotional states. Checking behaviors, counting, or ritualized movement patterns function to avoid or suppress perceived threat (Frank & Davidson, 2014).

Overarching Concept of Experiential Avoidance

Experiential avoidance is an overarching avoidance construct developed in the context of the ACT approach by Hayes and colleagues (1996). It describes the attempt to prevent contact with certain dimensions of experience (physical sensations, feelings, thoughts, memories) in its form or intensity – even if this leads to more suffering.

When avoiding individual situations (e.g., flying), it is necessary to explore in more detail whether the person is avoiding *thoughts* of crashing or death, not tolerating the *feelings of anxiety*, or fearing *physical reactions* or *evaluation from others* who notice their anxiety. Attempting to avoid painful sensations limits the behavioral repertoire and disconnects the person from important feedback loops, creates more problems, prevents accomplishment of important life tasks, and intensifies the experience from which affected individuals seek to escape (Hayes et al., 1996).

4.3.2 Cognitive Core Processes

The definition of cognition (thinking) goes back to Neisser (1994), who uses the term cognition to refer to all information-processing processes that process, reduce, elaborate, store, retrieve, and use sensory stimuli. Cognitive processes are central components of models explaining the development of emotional disorders (Sheppes et al., 2015). The thought process is dynamic and consists of an ongoing chain of information-processing steps. The ongoing thought processes generate constant change in conscious and unconscious mental states, thereby reinforcing or altering cognitive network linkages. Cognitions can be described from the perspective of their function as behavior or as a mental mechanism (De Houwer et al., 2018).

Selective Attention Focus

There is a wealth of research that supports the role of attention in maintaining psychopathology. Mentally healthy individuals manage to maintain an attentional focus that is favorable for coping, whereas people who have mental health problems often direct their attention to things that contribute to symptom reinforcement. These striking differences in attentional direction are evident across disorders. Empirically well documented and therefore worthy of consideration when analyzing possible problematic responses that cause psychopathology are (adapted from Harvey et al., 2009):
1. selective attention to external disorder-relevant stimuli,
2. selective attention to internal disorder-relevant stimuli, and
3. avoidance focus and attention focus on safety sources.

From a process-based perspective, these selective attentional processes can lead to unregulated build-up processes and downward spirals in which the threat stimulus attracts attention and further reinforces the threat character (Hayes et al., 2015). From a regulatory flexibility perspective, selective attentional focus fails to direct attention to targeted goal states as well as to take in relevant feedback information or use it to select appropriate coping strategies (Bonanno et al., 2004).

Harmful Thought Processes and Processes of Metacognitive Control

There are a number of generally harmful thought processes that (1) lead to fusion with unfavorable thoughts and thus promote inflexibility, (2) increase the effect of unfavorable thought content on emotional states, and (3) prevent functional regulation by their restriction to internal processes (Wells, 2009). These have already been described as vulnerability mechanisms; however, they can be observed as response mechanisms in stressful situations. These include cognitive avoidance through thought control, thought suppression and worrying, recursive thinking (in the sense of worrying as a process), rumination, and postevent processing phenomena (see Frank & Davidson, 2014; Harvey et al., 2009).

These cognitive response mechanisms are problematic because they create unproductive, self-reinforcing cycles. Repeated mental circling leads to a ramification and deepening of problematic thoughts and feelings instead of resolving them. Fighting worry with worry leads to a further increase in worry. Attempts to prohibit worry thoughts on the other hand also result in a reinforced worry cycle (Wells, 2009).

Cognitive Avoidance Through Thought Control and Thought Suppression

Cognitive control strategies can be classified under the domain of experiential avoidance (Hayes et al., 1996). Their function in the development and maintenance of various emotional disorders has been demonstrated primarily by the research groups led by Adrian Wells (2009) and Steven Hayes and colleagues (1996).

According to Wells (2009), the metacognitive belief that one can control unpleasant thoughts leads to an attempt to control or suppress thoughts. In reality, this attempt has a paradoxical effect and sets in motion a self-reinforcing, recursive process that leads to an increase in negative cognitive activity, an increase in fusion with feared emotional states, withdrawal behavior, and experiences of helplessness (Wells, 2009). This pathological process is also seen in individuals with PTSD. Negative appraisal of intrusions leads to attempts at suppression and situational avoidance. As a result, this increases emotional distress, increases internal arousal states, intrusion frequency, and prevents emotional processing (Steil & Ehlers, 2000).

Cognitive Avoidance Through Rumination and Worry

Worry and rumination can also be used as avoidance mechanisms in which the individual attempts to prevent other unpleasant mental images, somatic, or emotional activities. As a result, the attempt to apply brakes to a self-regulatory process disrupts functional emotional processing (Borkovec et al., 2004).

Worry refers to the threat of future events, so that repeated thinking through what may happen on a cognitive level reduces emotional engagement and supposedly buffers the aversive character. In reality, the prolonged worry process produces a paradoxical effect, increasing the intensity of worry and preventing adaptive coping causing further emotional distress (Wegner et al., 1987; Wells, 2009).

Rumination is a recursive cognitive process that relates to past events. It is controlled similarly to worry via positive and negative metacognitions and not infrequently serves cognitive, emotional, or situational avoidance (Wells, 2009). The rumination process is particularly well established for the development of generalized anxiety disorder (Borkovec et al., 2004; Wells, 2009) and depressive disorders (Wells, 2009).

Cognitive Fusion

Cognitive fusion has also been described previously as a vulnerability mechanism. Even if someone does not have a particular fusion tendency, cognitive fusion can be activated as a response mechanism. Wells (2009) has described the effect of fusion as a problematic process for the development of depression and anxiety, and in the ACT approach (Hayes et al., 2009) fusion is one of six core processes in the Hexaflex model explaining the development and maintenance of psychological suffering.

Cognitive Distortions

Cognitive distortions are specific situational cognitive biases, such as dichotomous thinking, personalizing, or mind-reading, and are activated by the presence of cognitive schemas. In Beck's (1967) hierarchical cognitive model, the schema "I'm not likable" can lead to having automatic thoughts in social situations similar to: "I probably did something wrong, surely the others will laugh at me." These automated responses are problematic because they reinforce underlying negative schemas and result in a negative cycle consisting of negative self-evaluations and avoidance behaviors (social and emotional) followed by renewed negative self-evaluations (Hayes et al., 2015).

Misattributions

Misattributions can also be very closely linked to vulnerability mechanisms, such as negative schemas or emotion regulation disorders. Thus, it can be difficult to distinguish between vulnerability and response mechanisms on a cognitive level, deciding whether the cognitive distortion is to be treated like a solidified trait (vulnerability) or has emerged as a response to an overwhelming demand the individual is trying to cope with. Responding with misattribution, by which the causes of negative events are internalized, results in negative self-evaluations and to feelings of guilt or shame. Automatic misattribution leading to enduring feelings of guilt and shame is a maintaining mechanism linked to the development of eating disorders, PTSD, addictions, anxiety, and depression (Stuewig et al., 2010).

4.3.3 Emotional Core Processes

Emotional Avoidance

If a prize were to be awarded for the response mechanism with the most major roles in the development and maintenance of mental disorders, emotion avoidance would make the short list. Many vulnerability mechanisms, such as deficits in arousal regulation, negative schemas, or impaired regulatory flexibility, cause individuals to have difficulty processing or enduring aversive emotional states. As a result, individuals are permanently confronted with difficult feelings they struggle to cope with. This makes reacting to these feelings in a way that prevents them from emerging or that makes them go away quickly understandable. If emotions feel unbearable due to low distress tolerance or are overwhelming because I have difficulty in regulating emotions, then avoidance strategies are the last resort. The problem with avoiding emotions is the same as with all avoidance strategies: It backfires and produces paradoxical effects. The feelings do not disappear but are merely postponed. Furthermore, burying one's head in the sand, when confronted with difficult feelings, blinds you to feedback loops and deprives you of learning experiences that can contribute to an expansion of your coping repertoire (Dixon & Rehfeldt, 2018; Frank & Davidson, 2014).

Hayes (2015) therefore suggests exposure-based procedures for depression treatment, as attempting to avoid unpleasant states contributes to reinforcement of these same feelings. Additionally, emotion avoidance prevents the development of adaptive emotion regulation strategies, disrupts feedback loops, and is thus illusory and detached from reality. The paradoxical effect of suppressing unpleasant emotional states as a regulatory strategy has been demonstrated for pain (Cioffi & Holloway, 1993), greed (Szasz et al., 2012), anger (Szasz et al., 2011), anxiety (Hofmann et al., 2009), and embarrassment in people with anxiety and mood disorders.

Dysfunctional Emotion Regulation Strategies

The emotion regulation process has already been described in detail in Section 4.2.2. Dysfunctional emotion regulation strategies are basically attempts to avoid or regulate unpleasant emotional states when functional "top-down" processes are not available. Examples of dysfunctional emotion regulation strategies include compulsions, eating disorder symptomatology, self-injury, dissociation, risk behaviors, substance-related and substance-independent (e.g., gaming, pornography) addictions that have the function to escape or override unpleasant emotional states.

4.3.4 Motivational Core Processes

In order to respond to demands, the maintenance and modulation of the motivational process is crucial. The vulnerability mechanisms described so far create resistance to change. Many of the response mechanisms outlined are avoidant or focused on enduring a maladaptive network state. In a maladaptive network, vulnerability processes, together with avoiding response mechanisms, form a relative balance in which the motivation for change is halted. So, although clients have a high treatment motivation, they normally display a low motivation to change. On a motivational level, the beginning of most therapies is not an ideal starting point to initiate a flexible, reality-based coping process (Berking & Kowalsky, 2012). Although the level of suffering and the desire to feel better is high at the beginning of therapy, avoidance and holding onto a stable state even if it causes suffering is also strong.

The motivation process was described by Prochaska and DiClemente (1983) as a dynamic process that passes through five phases (see Figure 33). In the *precontemplation phase* (*denial*), the problem is not perceived or accepted as a problem ("I don't drink too much"). In the *contemplation phase*, the individual begins to recognize the problem, and a *desire* to change something at some point is formed for the first time ("I should change my drinking habits"). In the *determination phase*, a *resolution* is made: "I will refrain from drinking altogether, even if it is hard." In the action phase, changes are put into practice (*implementation*), and in the following *maintenance phase*, changes are stabilized so that one does not fall back into old patterns. In the *termination phase*, the change is further stabilized and is felt as the new normal. This process is not linear: People may go through it several times and at times revert to an earlier phase. The motivational stage can also differ for different spheres in an overall change process. For example, if I decide to change my health-related behavior after a heart attack, I may be determined in regard to exercising more, but in complete denial with respect to eating habits. In this way the change process may seem inconsistent and contradictory from the outside.

By the time someone seeks psychotherapy, their own previous attempts have usually failed. Repeated failures impair motivation and lead to demoralization (Berking & Kowalsky, 2012). This explains why paradoxically help seekers do not believe they can be helped at the beginning of therapy. "I need help, but everything has failed so far and you won't be able to help me either" is the message many clients are sending in the first hours of therapy.

The motivation process is essential, because it controls, drives, or slows down all adaptation processes. It is therefore closely interwoven with processes at other system levels. In the context of the process-based approach, the motivation process determines the extent to which maladaptive system states can be overcome. To sustainably change from a solidified maladaptive state in a more favorable adaptive state, the motivation process needs to go through the following three stages.

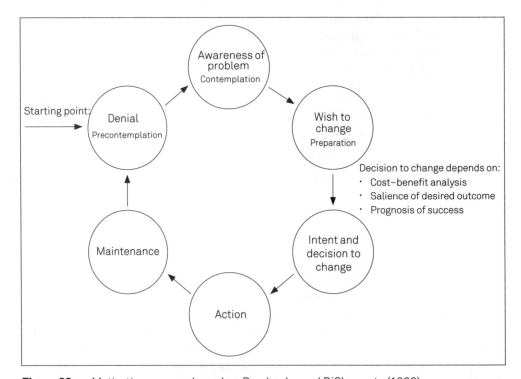

Figure 33.   Motivation process based on Prochaska and DiClemente (1983).

1. The relative balance of the pathological network (attractor state) needs to be overcome. That means the forces keeping the system stable need to be addressed to pass the tipping point of change in which the pathological network collapses. This means overcoming the avoidance motivation.
2. Destabilizing the initial network is not enough. In the next steps, the motivation process needs to be driven by an approach motivation (pull motivation). This motivation is not fueled by getting away from something aversive but directs actions and energy toward desired goals and consequences. This is a precondition for developing more flexible coping strategies.
3. In a final stage, the motivation process needs to transform to an enduring intrinsic motivation based on own values.

So, at first the client just wants the negative state to go away. "I don't want to be sad anymore" (avoidance motivation). In a second stage, the client directs their attention toward desired positive goals. "I want to be able be more active and feel myself again" (approach goal) and finally the person can connect with an underlying idealistic motive, securing an ongoing motivation to actively do good in the world ("I want to make a difference and contribute to the well-being of people around me").

Situation Orientation: Stuck in Enduring Wishing

Psychopathology, viewed as a complex network, is a relatively stable state. Psychotherapy serves to overcome this state and establish a more adaptive and flexible state. State orientation, in contrast to approach motivation, can be assessed using the energetic mountain-and-valley model of Scheffer and colleagues (2012) and Nelson and colleagues (2017) to visualize it. If sufficient motivation for change is not generated to overcome dysfunctional system state, the psychopathology will only change in the short term until the original state is reestablished. Most people are familiar with this phenomenon, when New Year resolutions to exercise more or eat healthier only last for a short time and one rolls back into old habits. From a motivational standpoint, we are in the contemplation phase or rather in the intention formation phase. In this phase of therapy, the client is in a state of "recognizing" the need to change or even desperately "wishing change" (see Figure 33). Both motivational states, however, do not yet generate a concrete motivation for change that leads to action. I have been desperately wishing I could speak Italian for 20 years, but although these motivation stages or recognizing and wishing are already reward-oriented and anticipatory, they are still passive (Berking & Kowalsky, 2012). It is not until the decision phase that this becomes a goal-directed "wanting" or resolution, in which the costs and benefits are related to the importance (salience) and probability of achieving the goal (Margraf & Berking, 2005). Before it gets real, my wish to speak Italian has to be transformed to the level of wanting to take lessons, deciding to learn vocabulary rather than to relax and commit to overcoming unrewarding phases in which I feel I'm not progressing.

In therapy, the client's "wish and desire for change" are often misinterpreted as "resolution." For example, an eating disorder client may report how much she suffers from malnutrition, how isolated she is and how much she wants to get healthy. "It's my biggest wish, believe me." Despite the strong verbal commitment, the client is still in the non-specific contemplation phase ("recognizing" and "wishing"). "Wishing" to get better does not necessarily initiate the desired change. Change is the result of an informed decision in combination with a specific action. Wishing to overcome an eating disorder is not the same as deciding to make difficult changes like gaining weight and being prepared to accept a changing body image.

Avoidance Motivation

As the previous explanations of problematic reaction mechanisms show, avoidance is a kind of "last resort" when attempts to cope with a situation remain unsuccessful. Avoidance motivation arises when a reward or a positive state is not sought as an approach goal ("pull" motivation), but negative states (punishment and displeasure) are to be avoided (Margraf & Berking, 2005). As described several times, avoidance motivation has little flexibility, low context sensitivity, and prevents adaptive learning processes.

Lack of Connection With Own Value Orientation

Intrinsic values are defined by Hayes and colleagues (2009) as the freely chosen, verbally constructed consequence of ongoing, dynamic activity that is intrinsically reinforcing in itself. That is, values-based activity is self-reinforcing, directional, and fulfilling. Intrinsic values are deeply anchored in cognitive-emotional schemas and intrinsically generate "pull" motivation. Values act as both a directional and a driving force. If attachment to one's values is missing, the person lacks this reinforcing drive from within and an important direction-giver. In this sense the lack of connection with own values is a vulnerability factor, but at the same time people can disconnect from their value base as a response to being confronted with a demanding situation. This then promotes the development of depression and makes it difficult to adapt flexibly in the difficult situation. Since values, similar to a compass, only provide direction for our behaviors, but not specific steps, values-based activity allows for a high degree of flexibility. This overarching reinforcer and compass helps tolerate aversive consequences and resistance (Bennett & Oliver, 2019).

4.3.5 Social and Interpersonal Processes

The processes presented so far focus strongly on the intrapersonal regulation process. However, the human being is a social being. The desire for connectedness with others is a central basic need of most people and others are a source for help when confronted with difficult external or internal states.

Interactions Between Interpersonal Factors and Psychopathology

Interpersonal deficits can be a vulnerability mechanism by contributing to conflict or disruption in relationships, which can then promote the development of mental disorders. Lack of interpersonal skills can limit the use of social resources and coping strategies. Conversely, mental illness can have a negative effect on the ability to form and maintain relationships, leading to isolation and loneliness.

Using social support is in itself an important regulatory strategy. Social support can be instrumental (e.g., material things), informational ("What did you do in that situation?"), or emotional (comfort, understanding). Interpersonal emotion regulation is thought to influence well-being, and social support is the medium through which interpersonal regulation is experienced (Marroquín, 2011).

Interpersonal Regulation Processes

Interpersonal processes can support a regulation process (be adaptive) or be maladaptive. A person with panic disorder who regulates their anxiety by taking their partner everywhere as a safety person is choosing a maladaptive strategy in the clinical sense, because it contributes to the maintenance of anxiety. For the process-based approach, this means that core interpersonal processes can trigger and maintain the development of mental disorders. The inability to use interpersonal resources for coping can also be a limiting factor in therapy. In contrast, the activation and use of interpersonal resources may be central to the development of an adaptive coping network. Thus, the process-based approach broadens the perspective to interpersonal factors and places them on an equal footing with intrapersonal aspects.

5
Psychotherapy From a Process-Based Perspective

5.1 Core Processes of Psychotherapy

Process-based psychotherapy aims to identify and change the relevant core biopsychosocial processes of an individual's pathological dynamics – for a *specific* person, in a *specific* situation, with a *specific* therapeutic goal. Therapeutic processes are the underlying mechanisms of change that lead to the achievement of desired therapeutic goals (Hofmann & Hayes, 2019).

The therapeutic process is:
1. Theoretically sound: The process is based on scientifically verifiable theories.
2. Dynamic and ongoing: The process involves feedback loops and nonlinear changes that are continuously evolving toward a desired goal.
3. Multidimensional or effective at different levels: Changes take place at different system levels (behavioral, emotional, cognitive, physiological) that interact with each other.
4. Goal-oriented: That is, change processes are focused on both an immediate and a long-term goal.

Klaus Grawe (1995; Grawe et al., 1994) worked to develop a scientifically based psychotherapy that focused on relevant processes of change rather than on diagnoses and therapeutic procedures. In doing so, he postulated four core factors of therapeutic change: resource activation, problem actualization, problem resolution, and motivational clarification. The significant thing about this approach was that he focused on the effective process of change and not on a therapy method. Through this approach, Klaus Grawe wanted to place psychotherapy on an overarching scientific foundation instead of confirming the supremacy of one therapy method over another. By focusing on identified processes of change in all therapies he sought to move psychotherapy away from belief systems toward a scientific-based profession.

Klaus Grawe was a forward thinker; the core factors he postulated originated in his "general psychotherapeutic theory of change." They were derived from a theory that had not yet been validated. In the meantime, numerous core processes of change have been empirically confirmed. In addition, several meta-analyses have been conducted to empirically prove effective factors of cognitive behavioral therapy (CBT) and third-wave methods. The most comprehensive work is by Kazantzis and colleagues (2018).

The following are essential for effective psychotherapy, according to the summary of reviews of existing meta-analyses by Kazantzis and colleagues (2018):

1. *Decoupling* from existing cognitive-emotional schemas (depending on the therapeutic background, one would speak of *decentering, defusion strategies, detached mindfulness, mindfulness methods,* or *self as context*).
2. Influencing cognitive processes, such as attentional focus and stopping unfavorable processes (e.g., fused recursive thinking, as in rumination, worrying, and negative self-referential thoughts).
3. The reevaluation and modification of thoughts and expectations relevant to the maintenance of pathological states (e.g., negative schemas).
4. The reduction of avoidance at all system levels through confrontation and exposure methods.
5. Improving emotion regulation skills (e.g., increasing stress tolerance, acceptance methods, habituation) and reducing dysfunctional emotion regulation attempts (e.g., suppression, avoidance, and self-harming behaviors).
6. The establishment of sustained motivation by aligning therapy goals with the client's value base. This establishes a persistent, self-reinforcing, flexible goal state as an approach goal. This contrasts with rigid, automated S-R associations and avoidance goals that dominate pathological states.
7. The basis is an absolute consensus regarding the disorder and therapy rationale. This creates a strong cooperation between the actors in psychotherapy and serves as a basis of trust that allows openness for therapeutic feedback loops.

A more detailed summary of the impact factors can be found in Section 11.1.1 (see Table 8).

The process-based approach focuses on the systematic application of these evidence-based therapeutic change processes and methods to modify the processes that generate a pathological network (Hayes & Hofmann, 2018a, 2018b; Stangier, 2019).

The analysis of effective therapeutic processes helps focus on evidence-based significant and influenceable processes in psychotherapy. These findings from the review by Kazantzis and colleagues (2018) are well compatible with complex network models of psychopathology (Hofmann et al., 2016), models of dynamic change processes in therapy (Hayes et al., 2015), and are consistent to empirically supported vulnerability and response mechanisms (Frank & Davidson, 2014; Harvey et al., 2009) targeted in the psychotherapy process.

5.2 Process-Based Therapeutic Stance

In the following sections we describe the therapeutic stance and the form of cooperation with the client, which makes it possible to carry out a therapy based on core processes. Process-based work is determined by the focus on the process level and an open therapeutic alliance, which helps making background processes recognizable both for the therapist and the client.

5.2.1 Capturing Complexity With All Perceptual Channels

At first glance, process-based work seems complex and technical. But especially when trying to grasp interactions of processes on a cognitive, emotional, and behavioral level, one must open oneself to a more holistic perception. On the therapeutic side, this requires an open, mindful "zoom-out" mode in which one tries to look past the content and perceive what other information is perceivable on emotional, interpersonal, motivational, and metacognitive levels.

For example, a client with severe depression initially talks about the multitude of strokes of fate that have made him depressed. On the content level, there is nothing but gloom and helplessness. Nevertheless, his gaze does not seem haggard; his eyes even radiate something lively. For all his listlessness, his voice seems committed, and when he talks about people close to him, one senses his attachment to them. If you put the "reception" not on the content but on the nonverbal signals, you see a complex, positive, and resourceful person who is merely buried under an avalanche of negative events. This kind of complexity can be grasped less rationally than intuitively with a holistic view of interpersonal information sources.

5.2.2 Collaborative Empiricism

This somewhat bulky term emphasizes two important components of CBT work that also apply to the process-based approach: empirical methods *combined with* a strong collaboration between therapist and client (Tee & Kazantzis, 2011). Collaborative empiricism refers to working together based on appreciation, interest, and empathic respectful curiosity in developing hypotheses and strategies to address problem areas. The psychotherapist's role is to provide empirical knowledge and evidence-based methods for this collaborative process. Without a secure trusting alliance between client and therapist, it will not be possible to understand often overwhelming and shameful emotional, cognitive, and behavioral dimensions of problems. This process of information gathering, assessment, and hypothesis development is transparent and actively involves the client, creating a continuous feedback loop between client and therapist (Frank & Davidson, 2014).

5.2.3 Informed Consent

The collaborative stance described in Section 5.2.2 is, like all psychotherapy, based on "informed consent" (American Psychological Association, 2016). Informed consent refers to the client's agreement, based on understanding, to follow the therapeutic rationale. This refers to both being informed, i.e., understanding which methods are to be used to achieve which changes (costs and benefits), and affirming the therapeutic measures.

Such agreement is the foundation for a positive therapeutic relationship. This correlates with the strength of the therapeutic alliance and higher therapy effects (Horvath & Bedi, 2002). If, like in many cases, at the beginning of therapy the pathological network needs to be destabilized, it is the therapeutic alliance that gives clients the security to endure the accompanying uncertainty. Particularly important in this regard is the prediction of expected unpleasant short-term effects the client may experience (costs) during the change process. Clients often have the expectation that therapy will seamlessly replace an unpleasant state with a more pleasant state. To explain the uphill-and-downhill model of Scheffer and colleagues (2012) and to discuss the bottlenecks on the different system levels is essential to prepare the client. Otherwise, the client will interpret the disruption and emotional tension that accompanies therapy, the intensity of unpleasant feelings, or the impulses to stop therapy as a sign that the therapy is not working. By predicting these accompanying irritating symptoms, they can be seen as an indication of the progress already made. For example, clients could be told the following:

> When we are working on relevant core processes to help you cope better, you will notice that feared feelings will increase, and you may even feel the urge to stop therapy. This is irritating for you because you might have just expected to get seamlessly better. When that happens, let me know because that's an indication that you're taking therapy seriously and making progress. The route out of misery might take us through a few dodgy areas before it starts to get better. But by doing this you are tackling the problems that brought you into therapy, rather than trying to avoid or mute them. That means you feel the distress better before you start to feel better.

This coordination between therapist and client is very important. Bordin (1979) highlighted the following points as significant for this: (1) clarity about the division of tasks between client and therapist, (2) a high level of agreement about desired therapeutic goals and expectations, and (3) the affective components of the therapeutic relationship.

If one engages in the network perspective, the transformational process that the client experiences is a continuously unsettling process. Maintaining trust in the process and the therapist, showing empathy and compassion, and strengthening the interpersonal connection are core processes of the joint change process.

I (M. S.) explain the importance of interpersonal connection to my clients using the following metaphor:

> Therapy is a bit like a mountain expedition. We will explore new spheres of life. For this we form a kind of "rope team." Instead of with a rope securing us, we are connected to each other through a kind of emotional rope. We will sometimes cross anxiety-provoking points, and I want to be aware – via our connectedness – how you are coping with new and sometimes unsettling experiences. For this, I have to rely on you to send me those signals, and you have to rely on me to hear them and respond to them. We have to practice that. We have to use small gestures to show each other that we're still at the same point, or jiggle the rope briefly if we drift apart. Please don't hesitate to signal me when something doesn't feel right.

5.2.4   The Therapist as a Person

Support in therapy can only be given if one involves oneself as a human being. McCullough (2003) speaks of "disciplined personal involvement," Linehan and colleagues (2007) speak of "radical genuineness" to describe how clients experience a high degree of genuine validation through self-opening and immediate, authentic responses from the therapist. When accompanying someone through existential and highly disturbing moments, a detached professional therapeutic role alone is not sufficient. In critical and relevant transformational moments it is not a client and a therapist who interact, but primarily two humans. In this sense, therapy is an encounter at eye level.

5.2.5 Dealing With Errors and Uncertainties

The complex and vulnerable work on core processes is never error free and includes moments of uncertainty on both sides (Frank & Davidson, 2014). As a metaphor for dealing with complexity, I (M. S.) use the image of learning how to surf:

> Difficult situations in life, when we feel the currents of emotions and thoughts are like high waves at sea can be frightening at times. In therapy we want to practice dealing with these unsettling waves and learn how to surf. We will try to catch the waves that will take us forward. We will probably end up in the water at first – in other words, we will make mistakes. The point is to keep getting on the board and over time get better at anticipating when which wave will hit us. Sometimes you'll be upset with me, sometimes I'll be upset with you. If we keep on learning ways to encounter these difficulties, we'll get better over time and hopefully you'll soon be enjoying tackling life demands without the help of a therapist.

According to Persons (1989), dealing with mistakes, such as admitting that one has not yet understood something, apologizing for mistakes, or making an effort to take care of relational ruptures, is a crucial process that moves the client and the therapy forward (see also Frank & Davidson, 2014). Therapists are an important role model, showing that psychological stability requires constant adjustment and engagement with "difficult stuff." The therapist is not the all-knowing one who is above all problems. In this way, a process-oriented "work in progress attitude" and the importance of adopting a metalevel is practiced in vivo in the therapeutic relationship.

5.2.6 Flexibility and Loyalty to the Common Treatment Rationale

Engaging with the client's individuality, the desire to see the world through the client's eyes, requires a high degree of flexibility on the part of the therapist. This flexibility is not to be confused with arbitrariness. Each therapy requires individual adaptation of treatment principles without abandoning the underlying treatment rationale. According to the results of the review of numerous meta-analyses by Kazantzis and colleagues (2018), the key efficacy factors of therapeutic interaction are (1) consensus regarding treatment goals and (2) collaboration regarding those treatment goals. All other efficacy factors are based on this treatment rationale. A high level of consensus with regard to the treatment rationale is therefore a necessary prerequisite for effective therapy.

The process-based approach offers flexibility and individuality for this purpose, as the disorder model refers to empirically proven vulnerability and response mechanisms, taking into account the individuality of response combinations and interaction effects. It thus represents a kind of "open-source" model that combines individual conditions of emergence with evidence-based treatment methods on a scientifically sound basis, thereby leaving therapists and clients sufficient room for creativity to solve the problems (Frank & Davidson, 2014).

5.3 Evaluation of Adaptivity Based on Evolutionary Principles

A question that often arises in clinical practice and is not easy to answer is: What is pathological or sick and what is healthy or functional? In terms of the process-based approach: How do I distinguish an adaptive strategy from a maladaptive one?

Box 2. Excursus: pragmatic truth

One approach to deal with the question of adaptivity is the concept of pragmatic truth. According to this concept, a behavior can only be understood by knowing its function and context. On the basis of the sole information that a person runs to the bathroom and vomits, it is not sufficient to classify the behavior in a clinical sense. Even a thought like, "I'm not good enough" may be a functional thought and not part of a depressive network in need of modification. It may be a realistic evaluation of one's competencies in a certain situation. Only when behavior is evaluated against the background of the context it is occurring in does its function becomes understandable. For example, in the case of the vomiting person, did the person accidentally swallow a toxic substance? Is it a bulimic client who was left alone briefly after eating? Or is it a client reliving traumatic memories during trauma exposure therapy? These examples show that there is no objective truth, but rather behavior can only be understood depending on the context.

Functional contextualism means that every behavior must be considered in the context in which it occurs. Each person behaves in the way that is best from their point of view. Behavior in that person's context has a function. "Functional" means that it "works" for the person.

In therapy, we are concerned with the relationship between an organism and its situational and historical context (Hayes et al., 2009). It is not about "right" or "wrong" but about helping people in a "pragmatic" way. In other words, it is about what works best in the best interest of the individual (Bennett & Oliver, 2019). To do this, it is important to have an informed basis for decision-making in order to promote a more functional orientation of client behavior.

A basis for the evaluation of *adaptivity* in clinical practice is provided by one of the most fundamental theories of all: the theory of evolution. This theory deals comprehensively with the question of which criteria determine the adaptivity, and thus the long-term survival advantage, of an individual, a group, or a structure. For a long time, evolutionary theory was concerned with genetic principles. The theories were used to explain how evolutionary principles led to the shaping of certain traits. Behavior and learning are now viewed as part of the evolutionary process, where not only genes (biology) influence behavior but, conversely, behavior alters biology through epigenetic mechanisms (Slavich & Cole, 2013). Human learning and adaptation processes are steps on the evolutionary ladder where variability, context sensitivity, and choice of response strategies determine the adaptivity of the organism (Hayes et al., 2018).

Evolutionary theory deals with the question of what favors adaptivity. Thus, the principles of evolutionary theory can be applied to psychotherapy: Psychotherapy helps to find more flexible solutions (variation), to make decisions that are favorable for the context in the long term (selection), and to maintain this learned adaptation. In a sense, the clients seeking therapeutic help have strayed from a favorable evolutionary path and in therapy are using external help to get back on an evolutionary path that promises more favorable long-term consequences.

Adaptivity in the context of evolutionary theory is multidimensional, as the organism responds with numerous subsystems that must be coordinated (cognitive, emotional, behavioral, motivational processes, etc.). Evolutionary theory can be summarized in terms of a few central principles, which we will present below in a simplified manner so they can be applied to clinical practice. These are the four principles of *variability*, *selection*, *retention*, and *context*. In addition, the *physiological* and *social/cultural levels* will be included in the consideration of adaptivity (these will be referred to as levels of analysis in the following sections).

5.3.1 Variability

Variability is the core dimension of evolution. Evolutionary theory was initially concerned with blind genetic variability, which means that starting points are random genetic variations and it becomes apparent in retrospect which variation confers a survival advantage. The variations are therefore "blind" with respect to their subsequent advantage. Evolvability – the possibility of evolving – has now been recognized as an evolutionary principle. From this perspective, processes such as rumination, experience avoidance, low self-control, or withdrawal have little variability. Many of the vulnerability factors and psychopathological response mechanisms listed in Chapter 5 lead to more rigidity, narrowing of the response repertoire, less context sensitivity, disconnection from feedback loops, and thus less flexible adaptation (Hayes et al., 2018). Nethertheless processes like brooding that lack variability have not been sorted out by evolution, so apparently there are situation in which little variability is of advantage. It is about using variability at the right level to keep on track to desired long-term goals.

Questions that can be asked in clinical practice regarding variability are: Is a lack of variability in respect to a certain dimension problematic or an advantage in the given context? Does the chosen approach to demands lead to an increase in flexibility or is the response constricting? Does the response promote learning and growth? Is it focused on desired target states or only on avoiding aversive consequences? By asking these questions, we are trying to find out which responses of the individual are too inflexible to adapt. This helps us recognize on which level we can help our client try something new. In this sense, therapy aims at increasing variation, getting clients to try something new, and experiencing different – hopefully better – consequences. One client phrased it like this, "When I got stuck in life, I would freeze. Now I know it's not about knowing the answer to everything, but to keep on trying until I find a solution that brings me forward a bit."

5.3.2 Selection

In the context of genetic evolution, selection is initially related to the reproductive success of individuals or populations. It's about choosing the right responses to demands that ensure survival. Thus, selecting a response strategy is about considering the possible short- and long-term consequences for the organism. From the point of view of behavior therapy, this mechanism is moderated via operant learning.

In process-based psychotherapy, the question is whether the choice of response modes is adapted to the current context and beneficial to the individual in the long term. Response modes, such as withdrawal tendencies, substance use, avoidance, and suppression of feelings, may be adaptive in a developmentally inhibiting and hostile context. However, in a safe environment, these responses mostly have the opposite effect and are therefore maladaptive. Thus, from a clinical-therapeutic point of view, the question arises whether the chosen strategy is useful in dealing with the demands on the organism in a specific context or whether other possible solutions would be better. It is not possible to generally define one coping strategy as adaptive and another as maladaptive, the same as it is not possible to name the best chess move. It depends on the context. In this sense, it is important to keep in mind that suppressing feelings and avoiding situations that are associated with negative feelings and dissociation strategies may be life-saving strategies in some hostile situations.

People with mental disorders are often fused with their perceptions and think that their response has no alternative. It can be helpful here to take a step back and write down all possible ways of reacting – no matter how absurd they sound at first. This provides a basis for choosing from various alternatives and selecting the most adaptive option.

5.3.3 Retention

Retention (maintenance or preservation) means that an achieved adaptive state should remain stable and not need permanent effort to maintain. If I learn vocabulary in a quick but superficial way, I will need to learn them again and again. This means low retention. Using visual techniques to anchor vocabulary in my memory more thoroughly on the other hand might need more effort at first but secure the new words without me ever having to actively recite them again. In therapy retention is achieved through practice, homework, establishing habits, and involving the social environment to anchor newly learned response mechanisms. An example for a comprehensible mechanism low on retention is suppressing unpleasant images after suffering from trauma. Even if it works out for some individuals it requires constantly screening for thoughts, feelings, and triggers to avoid and then suppressing them. This coping process requires constant energy and attention and explains why traumatized people often feel exhausted even if they withdraw from most activities. Internally they are very busy detecting and suppressing disturbing thoughts and feelings. Therefore, from an evolutionary point of view, it makes more sense to emotionally process aversive images, thoughts, and feelings even if this is at first very disrupting.

5.3.4 Context

Evolutionary principles are always contextual. It is always a matter of selecting the most adaptive response for the given context. This makes it clear that general, nomothetic strategies are often not context sensitive. For example, a psychotherapist may have discovered the benefits of a particular meditation technique for coping with difficult life situations. However, he should not transfer this strategy, which is highly effective for him, to a client from a completely different life context. In another context, meditation may seem alien or irritating.

5.3.5   Physiological and Social/Cultural Level of Analysis

When most people think of evolutionary theory, they usually think of selection by random genetic variability. However, evolutionary theory has since evolved and its principles have been applied to different levels to include genetic, epigenetic, behavioral, cognitive, emotional, and social processes.

In the clinical context, it is helpful to distinguish between the *physiological* and the *social/cultural* level. A reaction may be beneficial on an individual physiological level, e.g., to strictly separate oneself from demands of others in order to avoid stress. On a social level, however, this strategy may interfere with feelings of connectedness or isolate the individual from social support. In clinical practice, therefore, the issue is not only whether the strategy is effective for the individual, but also the impact on other spheres of life and the group to which the person belongs.

When working with anorexic clients, this often becomes an issue when the eating disorder does not cause intra-individual distress. The anorexic client "feels great," suffers few bodily symptoms, and achieves school or vocational demands. Affected young women may even seem proud of their discipline and low weight. By discussing the potential impact of the anorexic behavior on a social level, like the effect it has on partnership, friendships and family, these social costs become apparent (Hayes et al., 2018). On a social level, affected women can more easily anticipate and relate to the long-term consequences an eating disorder has. They can anticipate that the bubble of an eating disorder will exclude them from important social domains. The fear the family may collapse under the strain of the disorder or the sense of isolation and alienation despite appearing successful from an outside view is sometimes the main source of motivation to change.

5.3.6   Application of the Principles of Evolution in the Psychotherapeutic Context

The described four evolutionary principles *variability*, *selection*, *retention*, and *context* can provide us with guidance in psychotherapeutic practice to distinguish adaptive from less adaptive ways of responding for a given individual in a specific context (Hayes, Hofmann, & Ciarrochi, 2020). The "extended evolutionary meta-model" (Hayes & Hofmann, 2020; Hayes, Hofmann & Ciarrochi, 2020) arranges the four principles together with the following levels or dimensions in a matrix (see Worksheet 14: Assessment of Adaptivity; see Appendix and Section 10.2):

- System levels:
  - Emotion
  - Cognition
  - Attention
  - Self
  - Behavior
  - Motivation

- Levels of analysis:
  - Physiological
  - Social/cultural

To assess adaptivity, responses at each of the system levels, as well as the physiological and social/cultural levels, can each be assessed and evaluated using the four evolutionary principles or criteria. While attention and self are assigned to the cognitive level in this book, they represent independent levels or dimensions in the evolutionary meta-model. Discussing these criteria for assessing responses in a transparent manner can help guide therapeutic decisions.

After this theoretical introduction, in the second part we want to present the benefits of a process-focused CBT for practice in concrete terms and with examples from practice.

Part II

Applying the Process-Based Approach in Practice

6 Phases of Process-Based Psychotherapy

This second part of the book describes the practical application of the process-based concepts presented in the first part. We describe the phases of therapy and use practical examples to explain the process-based focus.

To understand the multilevel approach of process-based psychotherapy, a metaphor about demolishing buildings helps: A client's mental disorders are like a ramshackle, multistory building that you want to bring down with a few targeted interventions to make way for a more functional building (see Figure 34). However, one does not want to unsystematically bring down walls with global approaches. The question is: Which "walls," i.e., which processes, must one destabilize in order for the pathological construct to col-

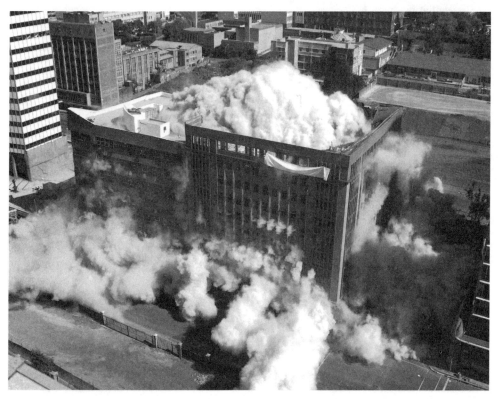

Figure 34. Analogy: A mental disorder is like a multistory building that needs to be brought down by deliberate and very targeted destabilizations (© iStock.com/BryanLever).

lapse? To obtain this information, a process-based disease model is created together with the client, which provides clues as to which processes are responsible for the stability of the present pathological network. The development of this complex, individual network model occupies a large space in the therapy. As for any evidence-based therapy, a differentiated understanding of the disorder also forms the foundation for the process-based therapeutic approach, on which interventions can be planned and implemented (Bieling & Kuyken, 2003).

According to Frank and Davidson (2014), from a transdiagnostic perspective the therapeutic process of diagnosis, intervention planning, and implementation is an ongoing, hypothesis-driven process. Figure 35 maps this ongoing process of process-based psychotherapy into six phases of therapy. In the following, a brief overview of the content of each phase is first provided. In Chapters 8–13, the process-based procedure is described step by step on the basis of these six phases.

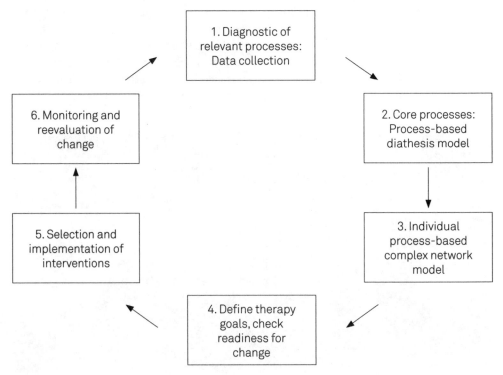

Figure 35. Schematic flow of process-based diagnostics, intervention planning, and therapy.

Phase 1: Multidimensional Diagnostic of Relevant Processes

The aim of process-based psychotherapy is to identify and influence the relevant core processes of human suffering. Most of these processes are not directly observable and clients are rarely aware of the processes causing the dynamics of their sorrow. That means relevant processes can only be identified indirectly by their effects and through observing recurring patterns. For example, a client may not be aware that focusing attention toward painful body regions contributes to an enhanced pain perception, or a depressed person may not realize that the constant attempt to determine causes for the depressive mood contributes to maintaining the depressive state. But, knowing what to look out for, the process-based therapist will notice that the client suffering from chronic pain attention is permanently monitoring the level of pain and in the case of the depressed client the therapist may notice the recurring preoccupation with the questions like: "Where does my depression come from? What is the underlying cause? Why me?" These questions, however, lead to feeling more helpless and guilty.

In order to be able to discover the core processes you need a broad data basis. It is like looking for gold nuggets in a riverbed. You have to wash a lot of mud and rubble, to find the precious nuggets. Because we are looking for the elements of a multidimensional process model, naturally the collected data should be *multidimensional, multimodal, contextually integrated*, and account for variation across the *time axis* (Gloster & Karekla, 2020; Hayes, Hofmann, & Ciarrochi, 2020; see Figure 36). The variations provide important clues to underlying processes responsible for these variations. This first step is by far the most time-consuming part of a process-based therapy.

In order to obtain this data basis, all available information on cognitive, emotional, behavioral, physical, interpersonal, and motivational processes involved is collected. Less attention is paid to the content of these dimensions than to the process. It is not what someone thinks that is important but how they think and deal with thoughts. In order to distance oneself from the content, it is helpful to generate information not only from verbal statements of the client, but to use as many sources of information as possible: In addition to self-statements, external medical histories, assessment of psychopathology, and behavioral observations, special process-oriented diagnostic methods are used to keep focused on processes. The longitudinal process focuses on multiple system levels and reveals recurrent core processes of psychopathology (Gloster & Karekla, 2020). In a nutshell, process-based psychotherapy consists largely of pattern recognition.

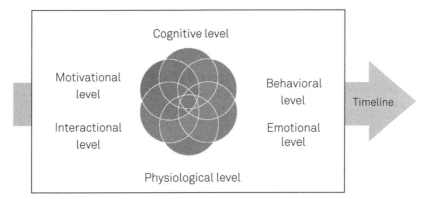

Figure 36. Processes become visible through longitudinal observation of variation at multiple system levels.

Phase 2: Core Processes: Creating a Process-Based Diathesis Model

In the second phase of therapy, the identified individual core processes of psychopathology are combined into a hypothetical process-based diathesis model. This model explains *which* core processes are involved in the maintenance of the observed psychopathology. Figure 37 shows a process-based diathesis model. The individual components have already been explained in Section 3.2.

This model reveals a first selection of identified core processes that may play a role in causing a person to suffer. However, it does not yet describe *how* these processes interact with each other and how these interactions at the process level maintain the disorders, problems, and distress. These interactions are analyzed and dynamics are revealed in the next phase of therapy, when these processes are used to develop a complex network model.

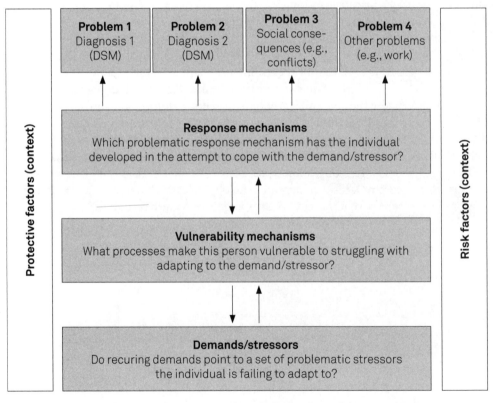

Figure 37. General scheme for a process-based diathesis model.

Phase 3: Developing an Individual Process-Based Complex Network Model

This individual complexity is taken into account in the third phase of therapy. In this phase the therapist and client investigate which interactions between core processes develop a sustaining dynamic in this person. The result is a complex network model based on processes. Its creation is described in more detail in Chapter 10. Figure 38 shows an example of a complex network model of a depressed client. Crucial in this network model are the interactions between the processes, which are shown as arrows of different thickness. For the same diagnosis, different process dimensions (boxes) can create a depressive network, and even when the core processes (boxes) are the same, other interactions (arrows) may be responsible for maintaining the disorder.

In this depressed client, the negative affect (as vulnerability) and the rumination reaction used to avoid negative feelings reinforce each other. For this client, the initial separation from his partner is particularly problematic because it activates an existing attachment disorder and thus generates more negative affect to the already high level of existing negative affect. At the same time, rumination is coupled with withdrawal behavior via self-reinforcing loops. The more the sufferer withdraws, the more he ruminates and vice versa. These two core avoidant processes create a downward spiral and contribute to the maintenance of his depressive state. At this level of analysis of an individualized process model, possible process goals become apparent to interrupt the perpetuating reinforcing spirals. The arrows in Figure 38 indicate the force fields relevant to the disorder. These are also the starting points for effective interventions to slow down the "flywheel" that the arrows create. Process goals in this case are (1) to reduce the intensity of rumination through defusion strategies, (2) to reduce withdrawal behavior through activation techniques, and (3) to decouple thought and action from negative affect. One can see the high individuality of the disorder model, explaining how two individuals with the same categorical diagnosis need not have process-level correspondence.

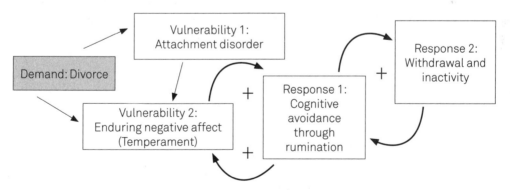

Figure 38. Example of a complex network model of a depressed client.

Phase 4: Defining Therapy Goals and Evaluating Readiness for Change

In the fourth phase of therapy, as in any therapy, *global* therapy goals are defined. Only when the network dynamics prevent the person concerned from achieving their global goals does a therapy assignment to change something make sense. Once the global goals are definable, concrete *process goals* can be derived from the network model. That is, what processes should change in the current network to overcome the pathological state and enable convergence toward the global therapy goals? The extended evolutionary meta-model described in Section 5.3.6 can help assess the adaptivity of previous ways of dealing with problems (Hayes, Hofmann, & Ciarrochi, 2020).

Even if the benefits of the desired change are obvious, a stable motivation to change is essential to permanently overcome a pathological network state. In addition to the core processes that led into a psychopathological state, the process-based approach is interested in the processes that generate change. Thus, fostering a proactive change motivation is always the accompanying strand in any therapeutic process aiming at developing more adaptive network structures. According to the motivation model of Prochaska and DiClemente (1983), in the early phases of therapy it is a matter of moving from a more passive treatment motivation to an action-oriented decision and finally to implementation (change motivation).

Phase 5: Selecting and Implementing Interventions

When the person's decision for specific changes is sufficiently stable, it is possible to derive interventions from the jointly developed complex network model and begin with implementing first steps toward the desired changes. Process-based interventions target processes in the network responsible for maintaining or accelerating problematic dynamics. Intervention points are therefore process loops disrupting adaptive regulation. These can be self-reinforcing cycles on a cognitive (e.g., rumination), emotional (e.g., avoidant handling of unpleasant feelings), or behavioral level (e.g., negative reinforcement by avoidance behavior). At the same time, the therapy tries to establish an alternative coping network, by mentalizing alternative attractor states and developing a coping repertoire to achieve these goals.

Phase 6: Monitoring and Reevaluation of the Perturbation Model

The therapy process designed in this way constantly provides new process information. Through permanent monitoring of changes and evaluation of the effects of therapy on psychopathology, the established hypotheses are continuously tested. Monitors are important feedback loops necessary for learning and developing adaptive adjustment responses. An everyday example makes it easy to understand the importance of objective feedback. If I want to learn to throw a basketball into a basketball basket, I receive quick feedback about the outcome in the form of visual feedback: Does the ball go into the hoop or does it hit the ring or the back wall? Without this visual feedback, it is impossible to change or improve my throwing skills. That is like practicing blindfolded. I could practice many hours a day, and I would thereby solidify my existing technique but not be able to improve my throwing accuracy.

In therapy, this works in a similar way: Exercise leads to an increase in competence if the person concerned receives continuous feedback. In the previous example of the depressed client (see Figure 38), affect (as mood on a visual analog scale) and the duration of brooding in hours could be monitored daily and related to a regularly recorded depression score. In this way, the individual could make a connection between the technique used (rumination) and the outcome (depressed mood getting better or worse) and thus learn to change the technique to achieve a different outcome. If the hypothetical network model shown in Figure 38 is correct, a reduction in rumination duration should also lead to a reduction in negative affect (duration or intensity). As a result, the overall depression score would also decrease. If this effect does not occur, the influence of other processes has not been sufficiently taken into account. The network model would have to be adjusted.

In the next chapters, the individual phases of the process-based approach are described in more detail. Knowledge of the standard procedure in cognitive behavioral therapy (CBT) is assumed.

7
Phase 1: Multidimensional Diagnostics of Relevant Processes

The starting point of process-based psychotherapy is – as in any therapy – collecting and establishing a multidimensional information basis for the diagnostic process. For this purpose, the following data sources are successively viewed through a process lens: (1) the spontaneously reported symptomatology from the client's perspective, (2) a more precise exploration of conditioning factors at the process level, (3) process-oriented functional analysis, (4) longitudinal analysis of the course of the symptomology, (5) treatment history, (6) an external perspective on the symptomology, and (7) a context analysis of protective and risk factors. In addition, (8) core processes related to psychopathology are assessed, and (9) specific methods to assess and measure longitudinal process information are applied. The aim is to extract the core processes of psychopathology relevant to the individual from the data collected in this way (see Figure 39).

The procedure is described below as a linear, definable sequence of therapy phases. In reality, the phases overlap. If the client is able to describe internal processes in a differ-

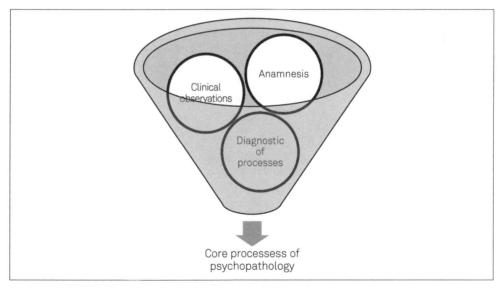

Figure 39. Core processes of psychopathology are extracted from the extensive data including the anamnesis of clinical history, clinical observations, and the diagnostic of processes.

entiated manner in the case history, some inquiries into a more precise exploration are unnecessary. For this reason, the therapy process depicted in Figure 35 shows a cycle: The therapy phases are passed through again and again, focusing on different aspects in each cycle, which are then combined to form an overall picture.

7.1 Spontaneously Reported Symptomatology: Recognizing Processes

From a process-based perspective, the client's narrative of what they are experiencing serves the process-oriented psychotherapist as a source of information in which processes become visible. The therapist observes how the client thinks, feels, relates, and acts. In doing so, they pay attention to what the narrative reveals beyond the content, such as how the person responds to demands in the world cognitively, emotionally, behaviorally, interactionally, and physically. What thought processes are triggered, and how is thinking controlled? What is the focus of attention? How are feelings perceived, evaluated, and regulated? Does the person have a repertoire to choose from or is the person confronted with problems empty handed? If different reactions to problems are available, does the person make good choices? How flexible is the person in their reactions, and how well are they adapted to the respective context? Worksheet 1 provides a guideline for process-focused anamnesis for this purpose (see Appendix).

Box 3.   Example: first utterances of a client

> **Therapist:** How can I help you?
>
> **Patient:** I am at the end of my tether. Actually, I needed this appointment last week. Now it may be too late. I've only been with my girlfriend for three months. When she messaged me last week saying she needed a weekend alone, it was another slap in the face. Out of the blue, she dumps me. I'm sure she's been cheating on me from the beginning. I was such an idiot to trust her. I got short of breath, thought I was going to die. I called her and I was beside myself. "Not with me!" I screamed. It felt so devastating. I got drunk, but it didn't help. I walked around the city all night. If she dumps me, I don't know what I'll do and whether I'm willing to stand that again. That's what I told her: "If you do that to me, you'll be sorry." She knows I'm not kidding about that. It's like this every time I get involved with someone. I hope you don't let me down! Most therapists won't even give me an appointment.

This brief introduction to therapy already provides numerous clues to possible processes that may be responsible for the emergence of the client's recurring problems. The narrative is like unfiltered raw material poured through an initial coarse process sieve. The sieve is knowledge of evidence-based vulnerability and response mechanisms, which were presented in detail in Part I.

This first "sifting" allows hypotheses to be formulated with regard to possible core processes. Worksheet 2 (hypothesis sheet on relevant core processes; see Figure 40, see Appendix) can be used for this purpose. Checklists are available for the targeted search for vulnerability and reaction mechanisms (see Worksheet 3 and Worksheet 4 in the Appendix). From the few spontaneous remarks in the above example, it is thus possible to filter out assumptions about presumed processes involved, which are summarized in Figure 40. This step is an incomplete and preliminary collection of *possible* processes. These may turn out to be incorrect or irrelevant in further phases of therapy.

This example illustrates that a few bits of information scattered at the beginning of a first encounter can provide a wealth of process information. The therapist's task in this early phase of therapy is to obtain as spontaneous and open problem descriptions as possible through a supportive therapeutic stance and to sort the obtained information according to the different system levels and the categories of the process-based diathesis model (e.g., external and internal demands, vulnerability and response mechanisms).

Once the client has presented their subjective experience, the blanks in the model are filled in by a more precise exploration, and the process of falsifying the hypotheses begins.

7.2 Specified Exploration of Conditional Factors at the Process Level

Based on these first pieces of the puzzle, it is possible to search more specifically for further demands or situations the person is struggling with and for repetitive vulnerability and response mechanisms by means of a more specific exploration. The purpose of the targeted exploration is to gain distance from the client's narrative and to obtain an overview on a more abstract level. While in spontaneously reported symptomatology the therapist follows the client's narrative, in this phase the therapist takes the lead and explores systematically according to the structure of the process-based diathesis model, filling the blanks and evaluating hypothesis. This is like a second sifting process: The information is again washed through the process sieve, and with each sifting process patterns emerge more clearly.

The following sections highlight questions that help detect external and internal demands and vulnerability and response mechanisms from a process-based perspective. Focusing on processes rather than distracting content is important because avoidance as a central feature of psychological disorders can otherwise obscure the uncovering of relevant response mechanisms. At the same time, it is important to explain each step in the therapy transparently, so that the client does not feel interrogated.

7.2.1 Exploring External Coping Demands (Threats)

People with problems can normally name situations that have caused, contributed to the development of, or at least triggered their problems. This sounds easy at first sight but turns out to be more complex when taking a second look. In the example described above, the client's girlfriend wanted to spend a weekend alone. Was spending the weekend alone the trigger here? Or was it the nature of the communication via text message? Or was the trigger being-prefaced-with-fact? Or were the problematic processes leading into a crisis triggered by the internal thought of being abandoned?

114 Chapter 7

Worksheet 2
Hypothesis Sheet on Relevant Core Processes

Demands/stressors	Vulnerability mechanisms (according to Worksheet 3)	Response mechanisms (according to Worksheet 4)	Consequences
External situation: *Partner wants to spend a weekend alone*	**Emotional level:** *Low distress tolerance Emotion regulation deficits Self-soothing and self-calming deficits*	**Emotional level:** *Impulsive reaction Low inhibition skills Dysfunctional coping (alcohol)*	**Short-term consequences:** *Conflict Aggression reduces anxiety Anticipating re-gaining control and proximity Concealing feelings of uncertainty*
	Cognitive level: *Fused with rigid negative beliefs/schemata on relation-ship, the self, the world, and self-efficacy Preoperational cognitive level (Piaget)*	**Cognitive level:** *Quick and strong fusion with thoughts Negative attention focus*	
Internal demand: *Anticipating being separated Regulating intensive and problematic feelings Regulating relationship needs and stressed attachment system*	**Behavioral level:** *Impulsive reactions Reactive – directed toward short-term goals, neglecting long-term outcomes*	**Behavioral level:** *Problematic problem-solving attempts Impulsive reactions, including aggressive behavior Self-harming and suicidal behavior*	**Long-term consequences:** *Enhancing conflicts in relationships Causing further problems through short-term strat-egies that backfire (alcohol, aggression) High tension resulting in panic, helplessness Activating attach-ment system with fear of repeated loss and loneliness Depressive mood*
	Interactional level: *Insecure attachment? Deficits in regulation of closeness and distance in relationships Empathy/perspective?*	**Interactional level:** *Lack of social competencies Withdrawal from others*	
	Somatic level: *Low self-calming and relaxa-tion skills*	**Somatic level:** *Further somatic activation instead of calming strategies*	

Context factors		
Protective factors: *One long-term friendship Open to psychotherapy and help*		**Risk factors:** *Little social support History of aggression with police involvement Financial difficulties*

Figure 40. Example of an initial collection of hypotheses about processes involved based on initial information from the case history. Context is the initial stage of a couple re-lationship after repeated separations. Blank version available in Worksheet 2.

This example illustrates that an external situation can elicit a wide range of internal de-mands on various system levels. But which one is relevant? The *relevant external demand* is the one by which the person *subjectively feels threatened*. In the described case, it was the expectation of being let down in the relationship and the anticipated abandonment by which the young man felt threatened.

It is not always easy to identify what it exactly is that triggers a feeling of threat. The following questions can help to identify the external demands in a situation.

Box 4. Questions about external triggers and demands

Introduction: I would first like to understand what it was exactly that was threatening and stressful for you in the situation we were talking about. Therefore, think again carefully: What was so threatening for you that it activated you emotionally and physically?
Questions:
- Up until what point did you feel fine?
- What was it exactly that pulled the rug out from under you in that situation? What exactly?
- What was threatening for you?
- What were you afraid could happen?
- What was the worst thing about the situation for you personally?
- What would others say contributed to your state?

In the case presented here, the client reported in response to these questions that he had never felt fine. This made it clear that the specific situation was not the problem alone, but a trigger for existing maladaptive emotional networks. He reported that his problems had started when he was 9 years old, and his mentally ill mother had suddenly left the family. After that, he had been disappointed in relationships over and over again. This was the strenuous theme of his life. When he received the message from his girlfriend, he was immediately sure that he would be abandoned again. Asked what others would say, he answered that he had often heard that he just didn't trust others and would scare other people away.

Common external demands are, as in this case: losses, separations, failed expectations, overwhelming changes, or anticipated failure. Mostly it is about threats to important internal representations of oneself (self-image) or the world (basic values/motives: security, control, connectedness, pleasure).

7.2.2 Understanding Internal Coping Demands

From a deeper understanding of external demands comes an understanding of resulting internal demands to the adaptive coping system. In our example, the external situation triggered the expectation of being abandoned. This posed an internal challenge to the young man's attachment system, his social competencies, and his emotion regulation system. This is what we understand as internal coping demand.

An internal coping demand can mainly affect *one* system level, e.g., you cannot tolerate the feelings that are triggered by a situation. Usually, however, *several* system levels or the interaction of system levels are affected when coping with emotionally demanding situations. For example, certain feelings or intensities of feelings may be overwhelming (emotional level), what is experienced may be incompatible with existing schemata about oneself and the world (cognitive level), or may exceed one's behavioral repertoire

116   **Chapter 7**

or interpersonal skills (behavioral level). A bottleneck at one system level is sufficient to send the coping apparatus into unproductive process loops or to disrupt attempts to initiate coping responses at other system levels.

Often, sufferers focus solely on the external situation and find it difficult to shift their attention to resulting internal coping demands. It is often easier to complain about the (external) working conditions or characteristics of the boss than to recognize that one has difficulties in dealing with uncertainties or own difficulties to calm oneself down in tense situations. The following questions can help shift your focus from external events to internal demands.

Box 5.   Questions about internal coping demands

Introduction: I can easily understand that these events are stressful, but I do not yet know what it is exactly that is internally stressing *you.* The same situation can be stressful to different people for different reasons. Therefore, I want to better understand what the events have set off in you.

Questions:
- What was the worst or most difficult thing for you in that situation?
- What hit you so hard?
- Which personal *values* have been violated by this?
- What were you afraid could happen?
- What *feelings* in particular did you struggle with?
- What *thoughts* did you find difficult to bear?
- What does this mean for you as a person – for your *self-image* or your *image of the world*?

With these questions, the therapist begins to understand the demands with which the coping system of the affected person is struggling. The young man mentioned earlier reported a fear of being abandoned and described an "unbearable" emotional pain. He struggles with this intense sense of annihilation and the image of being left "behind" or "thrown away," "like a helpless child forgotten at the rest stop." Even drinking a lot of alcohol doesn't make the unbearable pain go away, he said. He struggles with thoughts of hurting the person making him feel that way but recognizes that this would not reduce his feelings of pain but would just create more sorrow. As a result, his thoughts dwell on the possibilities of ridding himself of the emotional pain by destroying himself. These answers show the multidimensional demands the affected person has to deal with: He has to process intense feelings, sort out confusing thoughts, regulate interpersonal or attachment processes, and regulate processes concerning his "self." At the same time, the answers reveal vulnerability factors and insufficient response mechanisms in dealing with coping demands on the attachment and relationship system.

The next step is now to conduct targeted research into vulnerability mechanisms.

7.2.3   Identifying Vulnerability Mechanisms

While exploring internal coping demands with the client, their vulnerabilities become more apparent. The following exploration helps to deepen the search for individual vulnerabilities that may impair coping abilities.

Discussing individual vulnerability also directs attention to internal processes and how to deal with one's own vulnerabilities. Instead of focusing on the external situation (in the sense of, "Make sure my girlfriend doesn't leave me!"), the focus is directed to dealing with internal processes: "Help me deal with my insecurity about being left." In therapy it is mostly about changing internal processing, not changing external factors.

Box 6. Questions exploring vulnerability mechanisms

Introduction: What stresses someone can be very different for each person. One person has a hard time with intense feelings, someone else is quickly overwhelmed from conflicts or choosing the right way to react. I would like to understand which of your sore spots were touched by the triggering events.

Questions:
- What is so difficult about it for you? (*Squeeze the orange:* What exactly? Why is that difficult?)
- Which sore spot did the events hit? Certain feelings? Thoughts?
- What is it that makes the event so disturbing for you? Let me see it through your eyes.
- Can you recall similar situations that elicit similar feelings?

Using Worksheet 3 (Checklist: Vulnerability Mechanisms; see Appendix), suspected individual factors can be explored with the client for which there are indications in the medical history (e.g., emotion regulation disorder, learning difficulties at school). Vulnerability factors often pose a link between different problems or explain why a certain person repeatedly gets into the same sort of problems over the life span. In this sense they in a way link different problems together and make them understandable.

In the case of the young man, his insecure or disorganized attachment representation accounted for many of his difficulties in life. This overarching vulnerability factor explained difficulties in relationships, problems in coping with emotionally demanding situations at school and later at work, or his tendencies to break off contacts and avoid problematic situations rather than to seek solutions. Dwelling on the question of what the difficulties with the present situation had to do with him and what sore points had been hit, the young man was able to talk about the fact that his life had always been overshadowed by this feeling of abandonment since early childhood. He just cannot stand the associated pain anymore. In this way, the therapy moved away from the concrete situation and focused on processes mediating vulnerability and coping responses of a specific person in his context. On this basis, it is possible to move on a step further and explore the response mechanisms.

7.2.4 Identifying Problematic Response Mechanisms

The next step in the therapeutic process is to explore the problematic response mechanisms. While the already identified external demands and vulnerability mechanisms can only be influenced to a small extent, the way someone reacts to these demands can be influenced. Over time, people tend to develop reaction patterns that are typical for them. Some of the typical reaction patterns are more successful than others. Identifying the typical, problematic reaction mechanisms and understanding how they work is therefore the linchpin in therapy. Worksheet 4 (Checklist: Problematic Response Mechanisms; see Appendix) summarizes the most important empirically proven problematic response mechanisms so that they can be more easily recognized. In addition to questioning the clients, information gathered through observation, interviewing family members or analyzing the biography for typical response mechanisms can be helpful.

Box 7. Questions exploring problematic response mechanisms

Introduction: Before you came to me, you had already tried to cope with difficult situations.

Questions:
- How did you first react when confronted with the problematic situation?
- What other coping attempts have you come up with?
- Has anything you have done helped in any way?
- Have coping attempts failed or worsened the situation?
- Have you done anything to endure your problems?

By system level:
- What would others say about how you reacted (in *behavior*)?
- How did you deal with the stressful *feelings*?
- How did you deal with the stressful *thoughts*?
- How has your behavior toward others changed (*relationships*)?
- How did you respond to *physical* symptoms?

The disappointed young man, who feared being abandoned again, answered these questions as follows: He had tried to escape the crushing feelings through alcohol, speeding in his car, and roaming the city at night trying to exhaust himself. These coping attempts helped him reduce or avoid painful feelings and stopped him thinking. He reported that he wanted to be alone and felt the impulse to destroy something. He vowed not to let anyone get close to him again. In discussing similar distressing situations in his past, he recalled that as child when he felt abandoned and some had tried to comfort him, he would fight them off, run away, and hide. He could see that even as an adult he was still reacting in a similar way.

7.2.5 Understanding the Effects and Consequences

Finally, the events, the individual vulnerability and the coping attempts of the affected person have effects and consequences. One of them is that the affected person has started therapy. Therefore, at this point – following the standard procedure of cognitive behavioral therapy (CBT) – long-term and short-term effects and consequences need to be discussed.

7.3 Process-Oriented Functional Analyses

By analyzing the spontaneously reported symptomatology and a more precise exploration, a first framework for a preliminary process-based diathesis model has emerged. After this general overview, the next step is to "zoom in" on individual, concrete situations. This increases the degree of resolution of the observation, and other processes come to light.

7.3.1 Selecting Relevant Problematic Situations

In order to carry out a functional analysis, you need to select relevant problematic situations. Often clients have already named various problematic or distressing situations spontaneously, when explaining the development of certain symptoms. It makes sense to expand this list and to categorize the situations experienced as stressful according to the nature of the coping demands. In this way, situations that are externally very different can be clustered into prototypical demanding situations or so-called metaproblems. One student named exams, small talk at parties, shopping for clothes, and conversations with her mother about old school friends as difficult situations. These situations, which differed in content, had the common denominator "fear of not being good enough." By grouping them in this way, it is possible to group a variety of difficult situations under the metaproblem "situations in which I feel insufficient."

Grouping problems in this way feels relieving to clients, because they realize that even if they have difficulties in many different domains in life, in reality the problems are only variants of the same problem. These prototypical situations are suitable for analyzing typical response patterns on a process level.

7.3.2 Process-Based Functional Analysis

How to work out a functional analysis with the client is part of the standard procedure of CBT. In the process-based approach, the focus is more on the "how" questions (processes) than on the "what" questions (content). Instead of asking, "What were you thinking in that situation?" the questions of interest are, "How did your thinking change? How did you react to those thoughts? How long did you think about it? How did your thinking feel (fusion/defusion)? What did your repetitive thinking for two hours lead to?"

Worksheet 5 (Process-Based Functional Analysis: Questions; see the Appendix) is intended to help distinguish between the content and the processes of the reactions when functionally analyzing a problematic situation. In order to uncover relevant problematic response mechanisms, the checklist of Worksheet 4 can also be helpful here.

The detailed "zooming in" into the individual system levels contributes significantly to the understanding of the problem for both the therapist and the client. This is followed by zooming out with an analysis of the course of the disease over the life span (see Section 7.4).

This very down to earth way to visualize and monitor processes will hopefully be developed further some time in the future, so that we will eventually have standardized diagnostic procedures for measuring core transdiagnostic dimensions of psychopathology, as envisioned by the National Institute of Mental Health's (NIMH) comprehensive Research Domain Criteria (RDoC) project (Vaidyanathan et al., 2020). The aim of the NIMH initiative was to make testing and imaging methods available to measure vulnerability and response mechanisms on an ongoing dimensional basis, and ensure that this "live data" will generate a disease model that continuously simulates the impact of therapy, much like a weather model that continuously integrates current data to update the forecast. Since this is not yet the case, the following sections will now present the currently available, rather "shirtsleeve" possibilities to record and visualize process dimensions as synchronously as possible in longitudinal manner to provide dynamic data to support the diagnostic process.

Visualizing processes is the key to understanding complex systems. Dynamic changes in systems are difficult for us to comprehend. We always fall back into our more static and linear way of thinking. Like evaluating other complex interactions in dynamic systems (e.g., weather models, dynamic development of case numbers in a pandemic), curves and ratios help us assess the importance of certain underlying processes. In concrete terms, 6, 12, or 24 cases of a certain disease worldwide are not frightening. However, if one visualizes the process by means of a curve, the exponential character can be seen, which helps to understand the relevance of the contagion process. Therefore, it should be a goal in any therapy to visualize important core processes or their effects to help focus on core processes that reveal if a process is working functionally or derailing in some way.

7.10.1 Recording Emotion Regulation Processes

Initial Assessment of Emotion Regulation Ability

The method presented here for assessing the ability to regulate emotions is comparable to a stress electrocardiogram. The aim is to see how the client in focus reacts to emotional stress and especially observe how the regulation process unfolds and is managed afterwards. How high does the emotional tension rise, and in what period of time does self-soothing occur? Does this happen on its own and in adequate time? For this purpose, clients are asked to record the emotion process by rating the amount of experienced stress or tension in one of the next situations that trigger a strong emotional reaction. In this way we gather additional information on the potential stress triggers for this specific client. Sometimes it is a situation that would be a stressor for most people, sometimes it can, at first, be puzzling why a certain situation caused so much trouble. Alternatively, standard stress tests can be used (e.g., performance tasks) to elicit stress in therapy situation; the subsequent reaction is then monitored via a self-rating sheet.

For monitoring purposes, the clients are given a worksheet on which they can enter the intensity of the emotional reaction over the course of three hours (Worksheet 9; see Figure 44): on the x-axis, the time is divided into 5-minute sections, and on the y-axis, the subjective intensity of emotion is shown on a scale between 0 and 10. Figure 44 shows

7.4 Longitudinal Analysis of Symptom Development (Life Chart)

A "Life Chart" (Worksheet 6: Life Chart: Symptom Development Over the Life Span; see Appendix; see also Figure 41) can be used to depict the longitudinal development of the course of certain problems over the life span. This longitudinal visualization helps to adopt a metaperspective and makes other process interrelationships visible in comparison with the survey methods described so far. Clients enter the course of their psychological complaints as a line in a coordinate system on the worksheet. The x-axis serves as a time axis, depicting the client's age in years. The y-axis maps the perceived intensity of their symptom distress, suffering, or impact the pathology has on their well-being and functioning. As a simple variation, clients can be asked to plot the course of their psychopathology (e.g., depressiveness) over the life span. The upper range of the coordinate system on Worksheet 6 (7–10) indicates high levels of suffering or severe limitations due to psychopathology. The lower range (0–3) indicates that the disorder was present but was experienced as having no or very little distress. This takes into account the dimensional nature and variation across the life span.

In addition to mapping the course of a disorder according to *DSM* categories, it is possible to map other relevant symptomatology or influencing factors using a longitudinal visualization method. Dimensions that can be mapped in this way are: general extent of psychological distress, disorder-related distress, intensity of work-related stress, quality of partnership, intensity of conflicts, degree of physical impairment, distress due to somatic diseases, intensity of financial worries, development of body weight, sleep disturbances, experienced loneliness, PC or internet consumption, problematic alcohol or drug use or extent of social integration. The possibilities to visualize the development and variations of dimensions over the life span are manifold.

The Life Chart is suitable as homework and promotes the development of a metaperspective on one's own problems. Nevertheless, one should set initial reference points together with the client and check whether the person concerned is capable of adopting a metaperspective. Especially the classification of severity requires defining landmarks together. Sometimes patients need objective criteria to assess the severity of a dimension. Severity criteria can include behavioral information like being hospitalized, longer periods of sick leave at work, deteriorating sleep, or neglecting important activities. By identifying indicators of symptom severity, clients become aware of early warning signs of deteriorating mental health. In addition, it is helpful to divide the time axis into manageable phases by adding memorable life events, such as graduation from school, change of occupation, moves, marriage, births, using auxiliary lines on the x-axis.

Figure 41 shows an exemplary Life Chart of a client who was very fused with problems in her partnership, so we decided to visualize the intensity of the partnership conflicts (upper line) in addition to the depressiveness over the life span (lower line). It was interesting to note that the partnership was experienced as conflictual from the beginning and that depression developed with a somewhat temporal delay taking a comparable but time-lagged course. This indicated vulnerability factors in the area of relationship/interaction. Thus, it was clear that the depressive development was coupled to the handling of adaptation processes and demands in partnerships.

Box 8. Questions to ask when discussing the Life Chart

- How do you explain these fluctuations over the life span?
- What was different during this period when the symptomatology was less pronounced?
- What factors contributed to the curve rising so sharply, or to a reduction in suffering in this time period?
- What were you doing differently in less distressing (or more distressing) periods?
- What have you noticed? Do you recognize any patterns in the development of your symptoms over your life span?

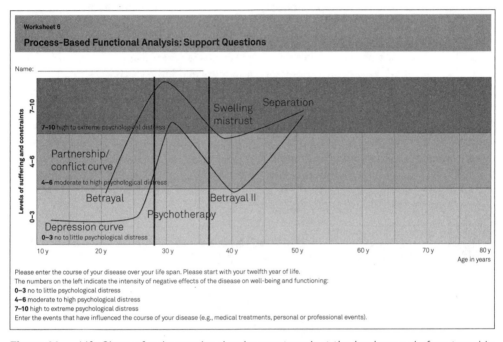

Figure 41. Life Chart of a depressive development against the background of partnership problems. Blank version available in Worksheet 6.

By visualizing the course of her depression and the intensity of perceived conflicts in her partnership, the above-mentioned client at first became aware that although being in a partnership was very important to her, it was also complicated and often stressful, and the quality of her partnership was closely linked to her emotional state. The Life Chart led her to look more closely at possible causal connections and she recognized that unsettling situations in the partnership triggered intense feelings of helplessness and initiated self-perpetuating loops ending in self-deprecation. This dynamic managed to kick off further depressive symptoms every time difficulties arose within the partnership. Her difficulty in dealing with partnership demands (vulnerability) in combination with unfavorable automatic response patterns triggered further symptoms, which together led into full-scale depressive episodes. After deducting this response pattern out of the Life Chart perspective, a major goal in therapy was to learn to decouple the unfavorable response patterns to insecurities and violations of expectations in the partnership and to replace the depressive, self-deprecating helplessness schemas with action-oriented competencies.

The Life Chart shown in Figure 42 illustrates the development of generalized anxiety disorder and depressive development. The client stated that she could remember being an anxious child, but as she got older she spent more and more time worrying. In her early twenties she can remember spending evenings at home ruminating about all sort of things and friends often telling her to stop worrying about everything. She was asked to retrospectively estimate how many hours a day she had spent ruminating in different stages of life. Although this is difficult to determine exactly, she was pretty sure it had gradually increased over time and she could remember lying in bed in the mornings or ruminating for longer periods in the afternoon, or not falling asleep because of her recursive thoughts. Over the years, the daily "ruminating time" had steadily increased from roughly 2.5 hours and had gone up to 7 to 8 hours a day at the time she started therapy. The first time she noticed that she was trapped in extensive worry cycles was at the age of 30 after the birth of her disabled child. While mostly worrying about the child, the worrying spread to other spheres of her life. At this time, she rated her generalized anxiety as a clinically relevant disorder herself. Retrospectively, the other depressive symptoms developed on from there as a result of her withdrawing from social contacts, giving herself the blame, and retreating from remaining positive activities. Plotting these different aspects of her pathology by estimating the hours spent ruminating retrospectively helped her realize that reacting to emotionally demanding situations through extensive thinking led to more ruminating

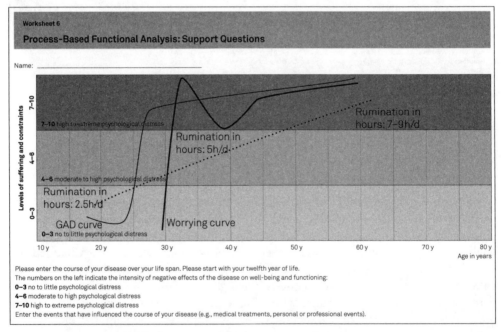

Figure 42. Example of a Life Chart: The course of generalized anxiety disorder and depression, the amount of worrying, and the amount of time spent brooding (hours per day) are plotted. Blank version available in Worksheet 6.

and merged into a negative spiral of worrying. Recursive thinking as the main response mechanism became the driving force behind the development and maintenance of the generalized anxiety, which in turn fueled the depressive symptoms. When asked what would happen if she could go back to worrying 2 to 2.5 hours throughout the day, she looked relieved and stated that would feel reasonable taking into account that she has a disabled child, but she would then have enough time and energy to live her life and she would no longer need to feel depressed. Metacognitive studies show that even healthy people spend about 2 hours a day ruminating or worrying about something throughout the day, mostly in short sequences of 20 to 30 minutes at a time. After that, healthy individuals note that this strategy is not working and they turn to something else. If the duration increases to more than 3 hours per day and the episodes of worry or brooding last longer than 20 to 30 minutes at a time, the likelihood of developing depression increases significantly. People are rigidly sticking to a strategy that is not working and therefore experiencing more and more exhausting helplessness.

Like in this case, a Life Chart can provide important clues to underlying core processes. However, there are also clients who are so highly fused with the content of their problems that they fail to develop a metaperspective on their problems. An example is shown in Figure 43, where the Life Chart consists of individual pieces of information mapped in a disorganized, chaotic manner. This Life Chart illustrates that external life demands are generally linked to extreme personal distress. Every life event seems to knock her down. This client's inability to change perspective and disconnect from the content of what happened limited the overall therapeutic process. This inability to abstract from the current

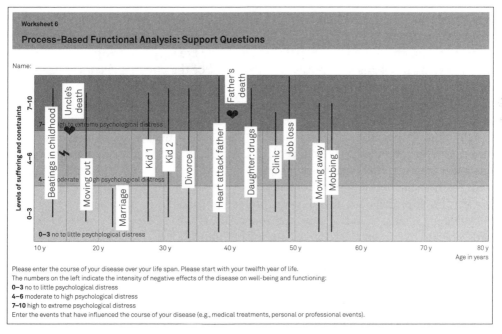

Figure 43.   Example of a chaotic Life Chart in which the client could not map the course of the symptomatology despite help. It is fused with individual events that are viewed independently of each other. Blank version available in Worksheet 6.

content was a core vulnerability process that explained why she had difficulties in coping in many spheres of life. As the examples show, the Life Chart is a multifaceted diagnostic tool that provides process information through taking a "view from space." This distant perspective reveals underlying recurrent patterns and connections.

7.5 Treatment History

The visualization by the Life Chart is also suitable for displaying treatments and treatment effects over time. For this purpose, the treatment times and relevant measures are also added to the chart. Visualizing the beginning and end of therapies, the use of medication or the use of other strategies shows connections between treatments and effects on the development of symptoms. The Life Chart in Figure 41 shows the period of the client's first outclient psychotherapy. The chart shows that, at first, suffering continued to rise during therapy. Suffering reached a turning point in the last third of the therapy, resulting in a decline of symptomatology. Recognizing these time-lagged interconnections is important because it helps to make correct predictions and build functional expectations about treatment effects.

7.6 Including External Perspectives

Family members, spouses and caregivers usually have broader and deeper insight into the problematic reactions of our client than we can gather by interviewing them in the context of a therapy session. Especially when clients are very fused with their perspective, analyzing problems solely "through the eyes" of the affected client can lead to a distorted assessment of the problem. Therefore, it is important to include an additional external perspective from people who experience the affected person in his natural environment. Assessing the external perspective is like another camera perspective that brings to light blind spots and details that the affected person is unable to perceive. Similar to the information provided by the affected person themselves, the information obtained in this way is "raw material" that must be viewed and evaluated through a process lens. Even if the relationship between our client and the external source is strained, their perspective may be helpful in understanding the problem.

Arguments against including family or close relatives in the diagnostic process are often: "I don't want to burden my relative with my problems," "I haven't let anyone in on my problems," "He doesn't understand me," or "She has so many problems herself." It is important to take these objections seriously and clarify that solving problems will require broadening your perspective. To give uncertain or dismissive clients more control over the situation, one can offer to predetermine the questions the interviewed person will be asked. Box 9 offers a compilation of questions to external sources to help gain an external perspective (see also Worksheet 7 in the Appendix).

Box 9. Questions to external sources (family, partners, close friends) to gain an external perspective

Thank you for taking the time to support our treatment. I do not want to bother you for long. I care very much about helping *<name of client>*. She/he has told me that your perceptions and thoughts may help us. Therefore, I would like to ask you a few questions.

1. How do you explain *<name>*'s psychological difficulties?
2. Until when was everything stable/okay from your point of view?
3. How did you first notice that something was wrong?
4. What situations do you think caused or triggered the problems?
5. How did *<name>* react to these triggering situations?
6. Have you noticed any changes in behavior since then?
7. Has *<name>*'s way of thinking changed?
8. Has *<name>*'s emotional state changed?
9. Has their relationship to you or with others changed?
10. What impact does the disorder have on you or others around you?
11. What would *<name>* need to change to deal with the difficulties?
12. Is there anything else you feel is important to mention?
13. Specific questions: ...
14. Do you have any questions?

These questions usually provide a wealth of additional information that complements the previous process-based disease model.

7.7 Context Analysis: Protective Factors and Risk Factors

Protective factors can lie within the person and – in a way – be the antithesis of existing vulnerability factors. Examples include a positive temperament, high flexibility, high insecurity tolerance, and stable self-esteem. Protective factors can also be external to the person, such as a supportive family. Effective protective factors in the social environment include: social support; a stable emotional relationship with a caregiver; an open, supportive family climate; family cohesion; models of positive coping; and positive friendship relationships (Bengel & Jerusalem, 2009). Basically, very individual aspects can make a person more resilient and buffer negative mental influences. The ability to be good or successful in an area of life (e.g., sports, music) can strengthen the experience of efficacy, self-worth, or connectedness to others, as can be seen in the following statement, "When I play music with others, I feel competent and connected to others."

From a network perspective, the use of protective factors activates adaptive network areas. One creates connecting points (attractor states) in a coping network, so that coping processes that are currently still weak have chances to establish themselves. A depressed client who had withdrawn from most areas of life was motivated to contact his former guitar teacher to take lessons. This one lesson a week did not change the overall depressive system, but the depressive network got a first crack by activating a protective factor.

Risk factors are, on the one hand, the absence of protective factors and all contextual factors that are associated with the violation of basic needs, i.e., security, control, and connectedness to others (Grawe, 1998). Examples include family violence, unemployment, chronic illness, poverty, migration, legal problems, mental illness in the family, and an environment that inhibits an individual's growth and development or is harmful (Bengel & Jerusalem, 2009).

When assessing risk and protective factors, a subjective rather than normative approach is necessary. For a self-confident, perfectionistic young girl with anorexia, the well-structured, achievement-oriented family system may be an additional risk factor, amplifying internal risk factors. The same family environment may, on the other hand, be a protective factor for her impulsive and less structured sister living in the same household.

From a network perspective, it does not matter whether the maintaining process is an internal or external. Therefore, influencing an external risk factor can be a key therapeutic goal to change the dynamics of a maladaptive network structure. It is often illuminating to explicitly ask the question about protective and risk factors.

Box 10. Questions about risk and protective factors

Internal and external risk factors
- What external factors have contributed to the development of your problems?
- What internal limitations prevent you from getting well?

Internal and external protective factors
- What abilities have contributed to your well-being despite your problems?
- What external factors have been helpful or kept you from getting worse?

When discussing protective factors, it is important to be open to whatever helps the client cope. In response to these questions about protective factors, one client replied that his deceased grandmother was in a spiritual sense always watching over him with a sense of faith and confidence in him and that this helps him through difficult situations. A 73-year-old client traumatized by an armed robbery reported that he had planted a tree as a child. When he was feeling bad, he visited this tree. The tree puts stressful events into perspective and gives him strength and confidence.

7.8 Process-Oriented Assessment of Psychopathology

Commonly, psychotherapists working in the context of psychiatric diagnosis-oriented settings describe the observed symptomology in line with common psychiatric symptoms. The Association for Methodology and Documentation in Psychiatry (AMDP) system (Guy & Ban, 1982) consists of a glossary of psychopathological symptoms (the AMDP manual) and several rating sheets. The characteristics listed by the AMDP system can be divided into two groups: psychological symptoms (100 symptoms plus 11 additional features) and somatic symptoms (40 symptoms plus 3 additional features). The focus is on neurological and psychiatric disorders and on the level of symptom. From a process-based perspective, this symptom-focused view is somewhat misleading and obscures the view of core cognitive, emotional, behavioral, somatic, and interpersonal processes of a disorder.

In contrast to psychiatric assessment of symptoms, a process-oriented psychopathological assessment directs the focus to the core processes described in Section 4. The findings of this process-oriented dimension help to sharpen the focus on problematic core processes and not to be distracted by symptoms that are in general a result of problematic processes. Instead of asking about the content of thoughts, process-based therapy elicits how much the person is fused with their thoughts, how reality-based or illusionary the thinking is, or whether the person is caught in unproductive thought loops. At the emotional level, not so much what is felt is of interest, but how feelings are perceived, how feelings are dealt with (avoidant, impulsive), and whether there are problems in emotion regulation. Worksheet 8 (see Appendix) can be used to assess core psychopathological processes.

7.9 Using Traditional Diagnostic Methods to Identify Relevant Processes

7.9.1 Established Test Procedures

For the field of diagnosis-oriented psychotherapy, there is a wealth of questionnaires that measure symptoms and symptom intensity. Many of these primarily disorder-specific questionnaires capture to a certain extent dimensions that can also provide relevant process information. One example is the Impact of Events Scale – Revised (IES-R) by Weiss and Marmar (1997), which captures the process dimensions of hyperarousal, intrusions, and avoidance. These three dimensions often represent core processes producing and maintaining PTSD symptomatology. The Eating Disorder Inventory-2 (Thiel et al., 1997) includes process dimensions that may be relevant for process-based diagnosis: Drive for Thinness, Bulimia, Body Dissatisfaction, Low Self-Esteem, Personal Alienation, Interpersonal Insecurity, Interpersonal Alienation, Interoceptive Deficits, Emotional Dysregulation, Perfectionism, Asceticism, and Maturity Fears. Provided the scales are sensitive to change, they can be used to capture core processes. Depending on your field of work, it may be worthwhile to evaluate the instruments used in your field of activity from a process-based perspective and to use those scales that operationalize the core processes of the disorder.

7.9.2 Questionnaires for Specific Process-Oriented Constructs

In addition, there are questionnaires that already focus on measuring general process dimensions of mental disorders. One example is the Multidimensional Perfectionism Scale (MFS-R) for measuring perfectionism by Frost and colleagues (1990). The scale captures the following four dimensions: *concerns over mistakes and doubts over actions, excessive concerns with parental expectations and evaluation, excessively high personal standards*, and *con-*

cern with precision, order and organization. Psychological flexibility as an important construct of the process-based approach can be measured with the Acceptance and Action II Questionnaire by Hoyer and Gloster (2013) or with the Flexibility Questionnaire by Benoy (2019).

Before relying on these instruments, one should carefully check whether a questionnaire really measures the process-based construct that one wants to capture. Flexibility in the process-based sense means not only variability, but also flexible adaptation to a context and the selection of an adaptive response that can be maintained (retention).

In the context of acceptance and commitment therapy (ACT) approaches, test procedures that capture core processes of the Hexaflex model are available online (www.contextualscience.org). The working group around Adrian Wells (www.mct-institute.co.uk) has developed numerous measurement instruments to capture metacognitive processes, such as the Thought Control Questionnaire (TKQ; Wells & Davies, 1994). Again, one should carefully consider whether the questionnaire is suitable for capturing a particular process dimension before using it: Beliefs about dealing with stressful thoughts should not be equated with the process of thought suppression.

As process-based approaches evolve, it will become more important to develop transdiagnostic, dimensional measures to objectify empirically documented core processes of psychopathology and change.

7.9.3 Neuropsychological Testing and Biofeedback Methods

Especially in the diagnosis of vulnerability factors, such as attention deficits, cognitive impairments or emotion regulation disorders, anamnestic information should be supplemented by objective measurements. With the help of neuropsychological test procedures, important vulnerability factors such as the ability to regulate attention, deficits in memory processing, and the maturity of executive functions can be assessed in a controlled and objective setting. If biofeedback methods are available, they can be used to measure tension regulation and to assess emotion regulation and self-soothing ability after being exposed to a stressor.

7.10 Further Process-Orientated Methods: Self-Observation and Visualization Instruments

Not all therapists have access to a comprehensive pool of standardized tests, neuropsychological, or biofeedback methods. In Sections 7.10.1 to 7.10.4, therefore, mainly self-observation and monitoring methods are presented which can be used to record relevant processes of disorder development without standardized tests. In general, the aim is to sensitize clients to relevant process dimensions (e.g., fused thinking mode during rumination). For this purpose, clients are asked to record this dimension as directly and promptly (synchronously) as possible on a documentation sheet over a defined period of time.

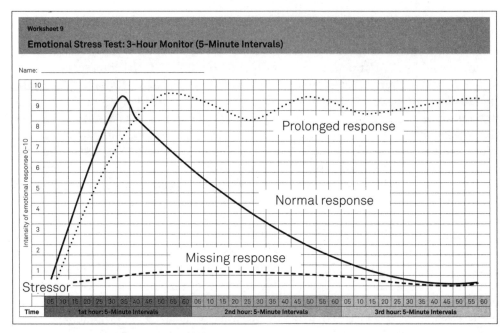

Figure 44. Emotional Stress Test: 3-hour monitor showing lack of reaction (bottom curve), a normal regulation to a strong stressor (middle curve), and a prolonged response (top curve) in which the individual does not manage to habituate. Blank version available in Worksheet 9.

three prototypical emotion regulation courses to a very strong stressor: a normal regulation, a prolonged reaction, and a course with a lack of emotional reactivity.

Normal Regulation of Emotions

When emotions are regulated normally, the curve shows a quick rise in tension until it reaches a peak, followed by a gradual cooling down phase typical to most emotion regulation processes. The curves differ in amplitude and duration according to the quality and intensity of the emotion the person is coping with. In a normal regulation process, self-soothing or habituation occurs within a reasonable time according to the stressor. In the hassle of normal daily life, the emotion may consume a person for 20 to 30 minutes before they gradually calm down and move on. If the event is really strong, like in an argument with a close person or when witnessing an accident, this calming down moment might take longer. In everyday life, depending on the intensity and quality of the emotional stress, this regulation process usually takes no more than 3 hours, so monitoring over this period is useful. For these individuals, the phrase "emotions come and go" is true. What is the appropriate curve? That depends on the individual factors of the situation, so the therapist's judgment is crucial to determine if the emotion regulation is normal. Clients should be asked to log the intensity of the emotion until they have calmed down, but for a maximum period of 3 hours. Many clients who come to therapy are convinced that something is wrong with their feelings and that they have an emotion regulation disorder. If one checks this hypothesis by observing emotion regulation, one often finds that the affected person has an appropriate emotional reaction, but they assume that "normal" people do not respond emotionally or at least are able to swiftly block unpleasant feelings when they occur. In this case, the regulation process is working fine, it's their expectancies and tolerance for intense feelings that is the problem. The monitoring of the regulation process therefore helps to discover and correct such misjudgments and rule out an emotion regulation disorder.

Emotion Regulation Disorder: Prolonged Reaction

Some clients, however, do not show an adequate habituation response after an intense emotional reaction. The intensity of feelings remains high or fluctuates in a high range of tension. To these clients the reassuring sentence: "Don't worry, feelings come and feelings go" is disconcerting as is does not reflect their own experience. The inability to habituate and show a calming reaction is not only irritating and unpleasant, but also has negative effects on the clients' cognitive, behavioral and interactional functioning. Experiencing how one's own regulation attempts fail makes you feel helpless and anxious, reduces self-efficacy, and also promotes avoidance reactions or the use of self-damaging emotion regulation strategies.

Lack of Emotional Reactivity

Some clients on the other hand show little response or no adequate response to stressors. They seem emotionally flat and unresponsive. They often return the monitor sheet and state that nothing really occurred to release a response. When discussing problematic situations, they report that their stress level did not really increase or at least they could hardly feel the difference. While many clients have too many intense emotions, these clients suffer from having to few emotions. Both extremes pose as a handicap when it comes to coping with complex and stressful situations. The lack of emotional responsivity may be related to a disorder in emotion perception, emotion building, or emotional reactivity. These individuals thus lack a central response dimension in the multidimensional adaptive apparatus, complicating the complex interplay between cognitive, emotional, behavioral, and interactional responses to environmental demands.

Emotion Monitoring Over the Course of the Day

The method described earlier gives indications of emotion regulation disorders in the narrower sense. The question then is: Does the emotional system respond to triggering demands adequately and are the experienced emotions processed, so that the emotional reaction subsides again? If this process of emotions surfacing and dissolving is functioning at this basal level, emotional difficulties must be sought at a higher level of processing. While emotion regulation deficits should be directly triggerable, other problems might only show in combination with other factors mediating processes that result in emotional distress. To capture these higher-level processes requires a longitudinal measurement that reveals reoccurring patterns over the course of the day or week.

Worksheet 10 can be used for a 24-hour assessment (emotion monitor over the course of the day; see Appendix, see Figure 45). Clients are asked to rate their emotional state

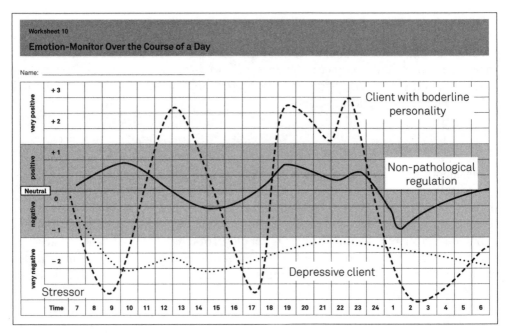

Figure 45. Emotion monitor over the course of the day: prototypical progressions. Blank version available in Worksheet 10.

every hour on a scale from –3 (*very strongly negative*) to +3 (*very strongly positive*). The zero line represents a neutral mood. Figure 45 shows three different curves as they prototypically occur in clients. The lower curve depicts the emotion course of a depressed person over 24 hours. The middle curve shows the mapped emotion curve of a person without an affective disorder. The third line shows strong fluctuations with high intensity in the positive and negative range. This curve showing the emotional ups and downs is from a younger client suffering from bulimia nervosa and a borderline disorder. Interestingly, many clients retrospectively map their emotional state at night because they perceive the intensity of emotions, thoughts, dreams, or a general tension even while at sleep.

Monitoring Emotions Over One Week (Emotion Protocol)

Another method of obtaining an overview of the variability of emotional processes over time is to ask clients to keep a simplified 24-hour emotion log over a period of one week. Worksheet 11 (emotion monitor for one week) can be used for this purpose (see Figure 45; see Appendix). On this worksheet, each line consists of 24 boxes, each representing 1 hour. The client is asked to mark at regular intervals (e.g., every few hours) the emotional state that is in the foreground for the past period. The more timely the logging, the better. Realistically, clients enter the values for the morning at noon, the afternoon values in the early evening, and before going to bed they assess the past evening hours. In the simplest variant, the client can be asked to distinguish between predominantly positive, negative, or neutral emotional states; for this purpose, the boxes can be colored in different colors (positive emotional state=green, negative state=red, neutral state=leave white).

Figure 46 shows such an emotion log or emotion monitor of a depressed client. The monitor reveals that the client already wakes up with a strong negative affect (dark gray boxes),

Example of logging positive, negative, and neutral affect states over the course of a day for the duration of a week. The worksheet shows:

Worksheet 11

Monitoring Emotions on a Daily Basis

Name: _____

For each hour, please mark the predominant emotional state:
negative affect/negative emotions = red; positive affect/positive emotions = green; neutral = white

Weekday															Time									
Monday	7	8	9	10	11	12	13	14	15	16	17	18	19	20	21	22	23	24	1	2	3	4	5	6
Tuesday	7	8	9	10	11	12	13	14	15	16	17	18	19	20	21	22	23	24	1	2	3	4	5	6
Wednesday	7	8	9	10	11	12	13	14	15	16	17	18	19	20	21	22	23	24	1	2	3	4	5	6
Thursday	7	8	9	10	11	12	13	14	15	16	17	18	19	20	21	22	23	24	1	2	3	4	5	6
Friday	7	8	9	10	11	12	13	14	15	16	17	18	19	20	21	22	23	24	1	2	3	4	5	6
_____	7	8	9	10	11	12	13	14	15	16	17	18	19	20	21	22	23	24	1	2	3	4	5	6
_____	7	8	9	10	11	12	13	14	15	16	17	18	19	20	21	22	23	24	1	2	3	4	5	6

Figure 46. Example of logging positive, negative, and neutral affect states over the course of a day for the duration of a week (negative affect = dark and medium gray, positive affect = light gray, neutral affect = white). Blank version avalablie in Worksheet 11.

and only distracting activities partially neutralize the mood (white boxes). Only a few situations in everyday life are associated with a change to a brief positive emotional state (light gray boxes). This client also experiences the night negatively. He sleeps only short sequences, ruminates, has nightmares, and lies tense awake in bed for long periods. Through visualization, the client often feels understood: "This is what my everyday life looks like – always trapped in depression, hardly any rays of hope." At the same time, the variation shows that the condition can be influenced.

When evaluating the emotion log, this client was able to determine that the few hours of positive affect occurred when in contact with other people. The most negative states occurred when he was alone. Also, over time, it was possible to replace the evaluation merely as negative or positive with the naming of more nuanced emotional qualities. The client learned to distinguish between "emptiness," "loneliness," and "self-deprecation" for the negative states (dark and medium gray areas), which he had initially uniformly labeled as "depressed" or "bad." Without reference to the monitor the client had described his depressed state in a completely fused manner as if he were in the middle of the depressed state speaking from within. Having the monitor sheet in his hands, he was able to look at the variations in mood from outside in a more detached perspective.

7.10.2 Recording Cognitive Processes

Monitoring cognitive processes is also about understanding how someone thinks, not what someone thinks. The most important construct in this context is cognitive fusion. This mode of thinking, in which one is fused with one's own thinking and can no longer view the thoughts as thoughts from the outside, is experienced as difficult to control and as limiting cognitive flexibility.

The first goal is to notice this not very helpful mode of thinking in contrast to a detached and flexible mode of thinking. Most people can describe how thinking changes when they get stuck in ruminative thoughts. Based on this, one can work out the difference between a fused and a defused thinking mode. Table 6 shows a list of characteristics worked out with a client to describe how thinking changes in each mode. It often helps to find a metaphor or image to illustrate the difference. One client reported that the fused thinking mode felt "like being in a trash compactor: It feels cramped, thinking gets tighter and tighter until you are crushed by your own thoughts." She remarked repeatedly in therapy, "Oh, my trash compactor has started. I'm using my strategies to get out of it."

Table 6. Thinking modes: Examples of characteristics of fusion and defusion

Fusion thinking mode	Defusion thinking mode
• I am fused with my own thoughts, clumped together.	• I am in contact with the world.
• It is exhausting, oppressive, rigid, absorbing, imprisoning.	• My thinking feels open and flexible.
• I feel I'm stuck in the middle of my thoughts.	• Thinking feels easy and does not cost energy.
• Thoughts block my view of the world.	• I can consider the thought as a thought.
• It's not me thinking, but my thoughts are in power of me.	• I can distinguish between thoughts and reality.
• I no longer perceive reality; it becomes more and more absorbing and abstruse.	• I can perceive my thoughts.
• A spiral that gets tighter and tighter.	• I can control my attention.
• My thoughts are narrowing my vision.	• Thinking feels agile and controllable.

A general 7-day monitor in the form of a simple log sheet is suitable for visualizing cognitive fusion (Worksheet 12; see Figure 47). The client can mark on this sheet, hour by hour, whether she is predominantly in a fused or defused thinking mode. In most cases, clients enter every few hours in which mode they were predominantly in the last few hours according to their own assessment. They then recall when one mode "flipped" into the other and are surprised that there are such different modes of thinking, influencing one's feelings and flexibility. At the same time, many clients make small notes above the boxes describing the particular situation, such as "alone in the apartment," "phone call from daughter," to record what was happening on the outside when the thinking mode changed.

Figure 47 shows an example of a monitor of a depressed client in early retirement who started ruminating as soon as he woke up. He stayed in his apartment most of the time,

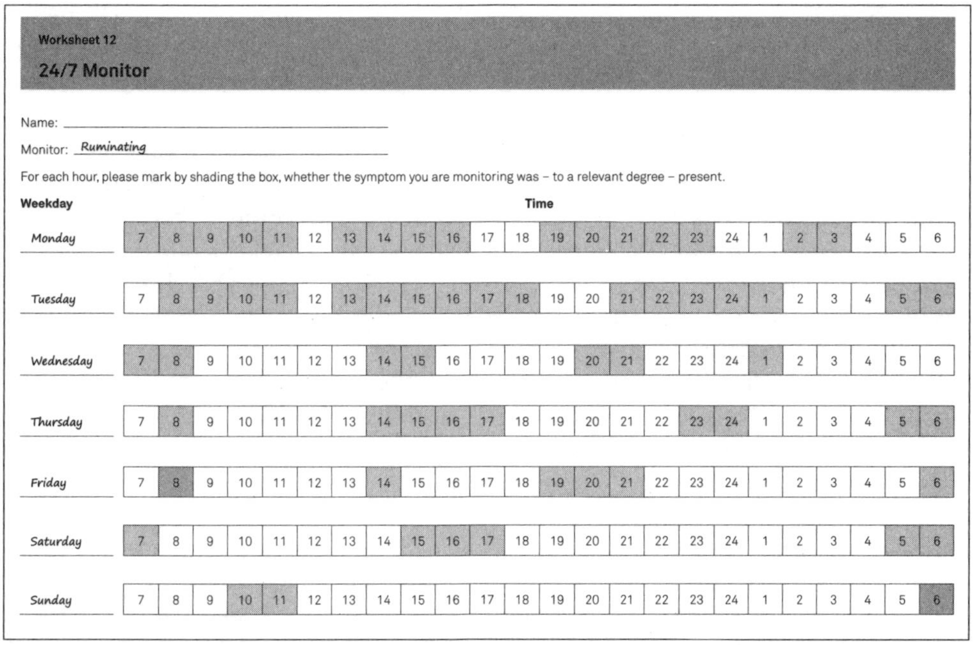

Figure 47. Example of a rumination monitor. The hours spent predominantly brooding are shaded. While on Monday the client spent approximately 17 hours ruminating, on Saturday rumination time has reduced to 6 hours. Monitoring symptoms often leads to a reduction due to raised awareness. Blank version avalablie in Worksheet 12.

thinking about his failures in life, and had very few contacts on normal days. Thus, over the course of a 10-hour day, a "fused-ruminating mode" accumulated. Problematically, this circular process led to more feelings of helplessness, negative affect, and withdrawal. This fused state was for short intervals, interrupted by activities, such as shopping or eating.

In many cases, simply monitoring the fused state already reduces this unfavorable thinking mode. Clients notice their worrying and rumination mode earlier, which makes it easier to prevent themselves from getting deeper into the problematic thought spiral. Asking "Is this thinking mode helpful in regards to your depressed state?" or "Would it have an effect if you succeeded in spending less time in this thinking mode?" sensitizes clients to the effects of fusion. Many are then interested in learning how to succeed in getting into a more mindful, detached thinking mode.

7.10.3 Recording Behavioral Processes

The general 7-day monitor (Worksheet 12) can also be adapted to record problematic behaviors. At the behavioral level, behaviors related to psychopathology are often swept under the carpet because clients are used to hiding or lying about these shame-associated behaviors in their everyday life. For example, in the treatment of eating disorders, the number of binging episodes, vomiting, the time spent eating, or time spent exercising are impor-

Chapter 7

tant variables to monitor. In the treatment of obsessive-compulsive disorders, clients are requested to record the time they are engaged in compulsive behaviors, and pathological gamblers may record times spent gambling or on the internet. The behavioral component is often quite easy to monitor, and it can be shocking what you miss as a therapist when you do not use a monitor technique and just rely on the verbal account of your client.

In the 7-day monitor of a client with bulimia nervosa, shown in Figure 48, the times at which bulimic eating attacks with vomiting occurred were recorded. This client was in denial in respect of the severity of her symptomatology, to herself and others, so the visualization helped here with a reality check and confronting her with a clear account of how the eating disorder had transformed her life.

This monitor revealed that she spends the biggest part of her day with bulimic episodes. She has to organize her daily life around these episodes, making sure it stays hidden from family and friends. The monitor acts as a baseline from which the effect of therapy takes off. Therapy targeted at a reduction of bulimic symptomatology can be tracked with the help of the monitor and assists clients to evaluate their progress. Directing the attention to feedback loops and ensuring that clients understand that it is not about doing the right thing but finding out what works and what doesn't by using feedback loops that is a core process in every learning process. Without functioning feedback loops, it's like practicing throwing a basketball into the hoop while blindfolded. You wouldn't get any feedback on whether you score, improve, or get worse. No matter how intensively and motivated you practice – without feedback on the result, practicing does not improve the trained ability. Constant feedback loops mirroring progress in therapy are therefore essential if we are aiming to improve the coping skills of our clients.

Worksheet 12

24/7 Monitor

Name: _____

Monitor: _Eating aattacks with vomiting_ _____

For each hour, please mark by shading the box, whether the symptom you are monitoring was – to a relevant degree – present.

Weekday — **Time**

Day	7	8	9	10	11	12	13	14	15	16	17	18	19	20	21	22	23	24	1	2	3	4	5	6
Monday	7	8	9	10	11	12	13	▦	▦	▦	17	18	19	20	21	▦	▦	▦	1	2	3	4	5	6
Tuesday	7	8	9	10	11	12	13	▦	▦	16	17	18	19	20	▦	▦	▦	▦	1	2	3	4	5	6
Wednesday	7	8	9	10	11	12	13	▦	▦	16	17	18	▦	▦	21	22	▦	▦	1	2	3	4	5	6
Thursday	7	8	9	10	11	12	13	14	15	16	17	18	19	▦	▦	▦	23	24	▦	2	3	4	5	6
Friday	7	8	9	10	11	12	13	▦	15	16	17	18	19	20	21	▦	▦	▦	1	2	3	4	5	6
Saturday	7	8	▦	▦	▦	12	▦	▦	15	16	▦	▦	19	20	▦	▦	23	24	▦	▦	▦	4	5	6
Sunday	7	8	9	▦	▦	▦	13	14	▦	▦	▦	18	19	20	▦	▦	23	24	1	2	3	4	5	6

Figure 48. Example of 24/7 monitor showing times of bulimic eating with vomiting shaded. Blank version avalablie in Worksheet 12.

In the case of the above-mentioned bulimic client, it was important to always use the monitor as starting point in each session to stay focused on the relevant symptomology and to counteract the denial and secrecy typical of eating disorders. Initially, she kept wanting to quickly put the monitor back in her pocket because she felt shame and guilt when her attention was drawn toward her problematic behavior. She felt more comfortable talking about more general problems, which led us away from the core processes of her problem. Changes occurred when we decided to focus on analyzing the monitor of her bulimic behavior since the last session and limit ourselves to elicit triggers and maintenance process of the recorded symptoms. The monitor became an active therapy tool she would point to, make notes, and plan alternatives strategies with.

7.10.4 Recording of Somatic Processes

The 7-day monitor can be used not only for cognitive, emotional, and behavioral processes, but also for recording somatic processes. Typical symptoms of interest in therapy are: weight, sleep duration, palpitations, pain, sweating, and dizziness. Sleep is a very general monitor that reflects the state of biopsychosocial self-regulatory mechanisms. Sleep disturbances are closely linked to many psychological disorders, and changing sleep quantity and quality can be an indicator for changes on other system levels.

Objectifying and visualizing symptoms, processes and modes help the client to recognize typical patterns and connections between variables and by doing this point to important core processes. Assessing these intercorrelations helps establish a causal model of the disorder. For example, a depressed client was asked: Do the hours of brooding and ruminating have anything to do with your mood? Is there a relationship between the number of hours you spend alone in your room and the hours you spend recycling your negative thoughts? What impact did your workout have on your emotional state? Although sufferers usually are aware that social withdrawal or rumination loops are conducive to depression, using a weekly log to monitor changes supports the assessment and change process and makes avoidance behavior more difficult.

8

Phase 2: Developing a Process-Based Diathesis Model

In the course of the diagnostic process described in Chapter 8, a wealth of multidimensional process information has been gathered. Anamnestic data were searched for relevant processes, situation analyses were conducted, the longitudinal development of symptoms was viewed from a metaperspective visualized with the help of a Life Chart, process-based psychopathology was assessed, and individual process dimensions were recorded with the aid of self-observation methods. On the basis of this extensive data, it is in the vast majority of cases possible to extract relevant core processes responsible for the onset and maintenance of the client's overall psychopathology. These core processes map the relationship between triggering problematic situations, individual vulnerability mechanisms and preferred response mechanisms. To complete the data collection phase, the identified core processes are arranged in a preliminary process-based diathesis model of the disorder (Worksheet 13: Process-Based Diathesis Model). This model then already explains what the eliciting demands or stressors to the organism are, which individual vulnerability factors make it too difficult for the client to cope, and which responses contribute to the development of individual's emotional distress.

The diathesis model shown in Figure 49 summarizes the essential core processes of a client suffering from anorexia nervosa and depression. Similar to other psychosocial consequences like dropping out of school or feeling isolated, the diagnoses according to *DSM* are under a process-based perspective merely the result of the interaction between vulnerability and response processes. It is not the illness according to *DSM* causing the other psychosocial consequences, but the processes unsuccessfully attempting to adapt to coping demands. The diathesis model shown in Figure 49 summarizes core processes that led a young student to seek help after dropping out of school due to her deteriorating body weight and mood. In the described case below we identified developmental tasks as eliciting problematic *demands*, such as accepting one's self (physically and psychologically) and dealing with uncertainty associated with growing up. These tasks were particularly difficult for this client because of existing *vulnerability mechanisms*: (1) a low tolerance for insecurity, (2) high perfectionism in different areas of life, and (3) a negative attention focus directed toward her "self." For this client, maintaining control was central. To do this, she used long-term *problematic response mechanisms* in the form of generalized avoidance responses or experiential avoidance: Referring to her body, she kept a tight diet, regimented her food, and divided it into good and bad food, and followed a daily exercise program of many hours. She avoided showing emotions, smiled away insecurities and fears, remained friendly-avoidant in conversation, and outwardly gave the appearance that "everything was fine." When asked in the initial interview how much of her mental energy she needed to feel so little and keep herself under control, she replied with a smile, "Over 90 %, and I can't stand that anymore." As a result, she fulfilled the criteria for the diagnosis anorexia nervosa and depression, felt socially isolated and dropped out of school.

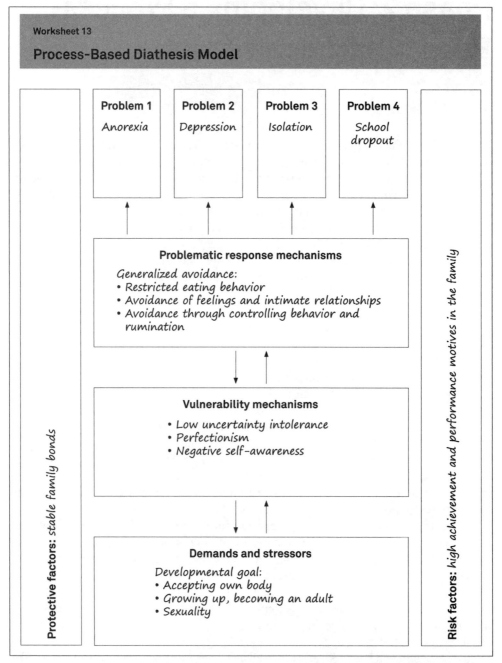

Figure 49. Example of a process-based diathesis model for a client with anorexia nervosa and depression. Blank version avalablie in Worksheet 13.

9
Phase 3: Developing an Individual Process-Based Complex Network Model

The previous diagnostic measures served as preliminary steps to get to the heart of the process-based approach: an individual process-based complex network model of the disorder. In the step that now follows, the identified core processes are put together to describe how core processes interact to create the individual problems of our client.

9.1 Practical Procedure for Developing a Complex Network Model

A complex network model can be viewed as a puzzle with interlinked elements giving both the client and the therapist a picture of the processes leading into one's problematic behavior and feelings and hopefully paths leading out of the distressing state. The prior phases of therapy have generated individual elements of a process-based diathesis model, which connects these elements through arrows visualizing dynamic relationships between these elements.

For the practical perspective, the client and the therapist discuss how the triggering situation interacts with the client's core vulnerability and problematic responses mechanisms causing psychological distress. It is best to note core processes on index cards and gradually develop a causal model, connecting each element via arrows indicating the causal direction. The therapist begins this process by noting a relevant trigger on an index card and placing it on the table. Further index cards representing core processes collected in the earlier stages of therapy are also spread on the table – like at the beginning of a puzzle. Taking a bird's-eye view helps the client step back and perceive the mechanisms behind his suffering. Using the triggering situation as a starting point, the therapist asks: "What does this situation trigger?" or "What other processes we have discussed and collected does the situation activate?" Selecting one core process after the other and asking how it relates to the other core processes of the model helps the therapist and the client understand the evolving dynamics of the interacting processes. This process is like picking up pieces of a puzzle and asking how and where they might fit in. With each piece, the picture becomes clearer until eventually a process model of the disorder is recognizable.

142   Chapter 9

For better clarity, different index card colors or shapes distinguishing between external situations, not changeable vulnerability factors and modifiable response mechanisms, can be helpful. Although I (M. S.) use index cards, therapists should use a method that works for them: Sketching the model on a piece of paper, using a flipchart, or using a digital solution like a mind-map or flowchart app have also been shown to be effective.

This process-oriented causal disease model can be used flexibly and individually. While developing a model, further aspects may arise and can be easily added. For example, in one case a client remembered that after reacting with withdrawal to a difficult situation her mother would get worried and call her, telling her how guilty she feels that her daughter cannot cope with life. This aspect triggered further problematic processes such as feelings of guilt and shame and was added in the course of developing a complex network model.

In order to be able to consider a certain interaction between individual elements in the disease model, it is sometimes necessary to give strongly interconnected process dimensions a more central position in the network, i.e., to move the corresponding card more to the center of the model. In this way, the model keeps changing its shape, and small subcenters with related network elements become visible. Often the model starts out looking more linear, becoming more and more like interconnected whirlwinds where dynamics are formed around certain central elements. After the intense phase of data collection, this phase focuses on understanding interactions and recognizing problematic automatic links between processes.

We recommend that therapists trained in cognitive behavioral therapy (CBT) first follow the familiar structure of functional analysis, i.e., start with triggers, consider vulnerability factors, and then add the various responses. This results in the sequence described in Box 11.

Box 11. Individual steps for developing an individual process-based complex network model

1. Determine triggering situation and internal demands to adapt to the situation.
2. Ask how individual vulnerabilities of the client hamper the attempts to adapt. Sometimes the combination of vulnerability factors cause the client to get stuck in the attempt to cope.
3. Identify the series of responses that the client activates as a result of getting stuck.
4. Indicate interactions (arrows) between the individual elements of the network model to illustrate how certain elements influence other reactions.
5. Consider other factors (contextual factors, protective factors or risk factors) maintaining the dynamics responsible for the clients suffering.
6. Include reinforcing feedback loops, like positive or negative reinforcement mechanisms.

It is not essential to slavishly follow the order of the steps described, because the complex network model is *not* based on a linear understanding. One client compared the procedure with a Sudoku puzzle, in which some elements are already given and one searches for the logical connection between them. In a similar way, the complex network model is completed piece by piece until it meets the client's experience. The individual steps listed are therefore to be regarded as points of reference. After working with process-based complex models for a while, one's own linear way of thinking slowly shifts to a more systemic understanding of psychopathology in which there is no clear beginning or set order. Psychopathology unfolds in a rather dynamic and nonlinear way – the processes leading in and out of a maladaptive mode have no clear beginning and no clear end.

The simplified example in Figure 50 serves as an illustration of a complex network of a client who sought help after losing a job. The starting point (1) is therefore the job loss. This becomes a clinically relevant trigger because it encounters significant vulnerability factors within the client: poor self-soothing skills (2) and a preexisting negative self-concept (3). Prior to the job loss, these two dimensions were not particularly significant in the client's life, as job recognition and structure in daily life were able to compensate for the negative effects of these vulnerabilities. However, the job loss activated these vulnerability mechanisms, so the negative self-concept in particular led to self-deprecation processes (4) that confirmed and reinforced the negative self-concept. These interactions are depicted by the arrows. Another problematic core process in this case is the client's attempt to "get a grip" by thinking intensively about his situation leading to endless rumination (5). By ruminating he repeatedly gets to the bottom of possible failures, thoughts of guilt, and causes for his failure. Instead of finding answers, more doubts and questions arise, which motivates him to think even more intensively. As a consequence, he loses himself in self-reinforcing loops that destroy the remnants of self-worth he still has. At the time of entering therapy, excessive, unproductive rumination had reinforced the effect of self-deprecation and produced the depressive symptoms, such as the experience of helplessness, sleep disorders, difficulty concentrating, and loss of self-esteem. These two loops visible in Figure 50 – on the one hand, the one between the rumination and the self-deprecation process, and, on the other hand, the self-reinforcing rumination process itself – are the engine that drives his depressive mental state. Recognizing which core processes drive the dynamics of the negative spiral the client feels stuck in helps direct interventions specifically to these maintaining factors. The job loss is not the problem but the previously described reaction and his inability to exit ineffective coping strategies.

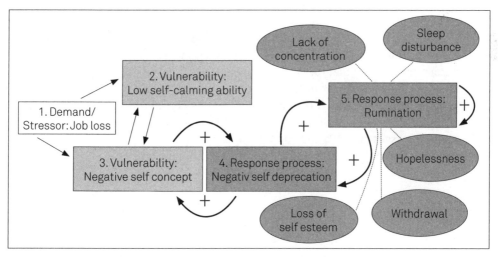

Figure 50. Complex network model of a depressed client with vulnerability mechanisms (light gray), problematic response mechanisms (dark gray), symptoms (ovals), and interactions (thick, curved arrows) that contribute to the maintenance of depressive symptomatology.

144   Chapter 9

This approach is more precise than a general depression treatment according to the guideline, which recommends medication, general activation, and restructuring of negative thoughts.

9.2   Evaluating the Adaptivity of Network Patterns Using the Extended Evolutionary Metamodel

Once a network model of the disorder has been successfully developed, work can begin with this model. The first question that arises is: How adaptive is the network model for the client? The quickest answer is usually obtained by asking the affected person if he would recommend his way of dealing with his situation to someone with similar problems. For example, the depressed client mentioned earlier might be asked, "Is it useful to spend 5 to 6 hours a day for months after a layoff thinking about your failures and mistakes and using them to validate your own inferiority? Would you recommend this in general?" A client with anorexia nervosa might be asked, with the network model in mind, if she would give a talk to schoolgirls recommending restrictive eating to cope with insecurities, or binge eating to get rid of intense feelings.

In Section 5.3, four different principles or criteria derived from evolutionary theory were presented for assessing adaptivity (variability, selection, retention, context). When discussing the network model, reviewing these evolutionary principles by means of Socratic dialogue can sensitize the person concerned to the maladaptiveness of their own ways of reacting.

9.2.1   Variability

Many vulnerability factors and psychopathological response mechanisms lead to greater rigidity, narrowing of the response repertoire, less context sensitivity, disconnection from feedback loops, and thus result in less flexible adaptation (Hayes et al., 2018). Bearing in mind that a central goal of therapy is to enhance psychological flexibility to enhance adaptive coping, the question to ask is: Is the current approach to solving external and internal demands flexible or rigid and confining? Does the chosen coping approach lead to more or less flexibility? Does it promote learning and growth or is the person merely enduring an unpleasant state? Is the coping response flexibly attracted to desired target states? Or is the client bracing to endure or avoid an aversive state?

9.2.2   Selection

Adaptive selection means choosing a response strategy by considering the individual and social long-term consequences. From the array of responses, there are not generally good and bad responses. Even in psychotherapy, we are sometimes narrow-minded and assume a certain strategy, like that expressing one's feelings or acceptance cannot be wrong. So, it can be helpful to ask: What other response strategies are available? Is the chosen response a good option in principle, but less helpful in this situation? Is the response perhaps selected because it has been effective in the past, but seems to be not working for the current situation? Often the selection is based on past experience and does not take into account changes in context or even current feedback. Like a traumatized client who repeatedly hid under the table with her hands in front of her face when triggered by intense memories of her trauma. Considering the many ways of dealing with an intense memory, this was a stigmatizing and very unfavorable selection. The client thus drew attention to herself and placed herself in a defenseless position in which her crouching posture with closed eyes intensified the intense feelings. Through a collection of alternative responses (including climbing on a cupboard), she was made aware of choices and the importance of wisely selecting her response, which gradually allowed for a change in the automated pattern.

9.2.3 Retention

Retention refers to the ability to maintain an adaptive process once established. Avoidance responses often lack this adaptive quality from an evolutionary perspective because avoidance is a very effortful process. It requires constant attention, monitoring, and thus energy to be maintained. Not wanting to think about something, not wanting to feel something, or not wanting to encounter someone requires that you constantly keep an internal representation of what you want to avoid activated. This does not satisfy the retention principle. This criterion is about checking whether the triggering demand has really been mastered or only postponed, avoided, or bypassed, requiring constant attention and energy-consuming devotion. This can be explained to clients well by means of a comparison with the backhand in tennis. For many, learning to return the ball with the backhand may be difficult at first, so alternatively you may decide to bypass it and hit balls with the forehand. This saves the effort and frustration of practicing the backhand. In the long run, however, playing with the backhand may be more energy efficient. Many clients quickly realize that they are bypassing numerous difficulties in their lives with high emotional costs. They often come to therapy when they realize that their approach to solving the demands is effective but not sustainable in the long term.

9.2.4 Context

Evolutionary principles are always contextual. Unfavorable adaptive responses are often directed toward a context one would like to *have*, not the *actual* context. To use a golf metaphor, you have to play the ball from where it lands (e.g., in the woods), not where you would like it to be or where it should be (e.g., on the green). This metaphor refers to perceiving the context realistically and accepting it. A client who was fired by her boss after giving honest feedback to her boss was confused because honesty and authenticity were important therapy goals. She had recognized that hiding her real feelings was maintaining her depressive feelings. In therapy, she had experienced the positive effects of being honest and speaking openly. However, she and her therapist had not yet integrated the contextual component. To analyze the adaptivity of existing ways of responding and intended changes in psychotherapy, the extended evolutionary metamodel (Hayes & Hofmann, 2020; Hayes, Hofmann, & Ciarrochi, 2020; see Section 5.3; see also Worksheet 14: Assessment of Adaptivity in the Appendix) can be helpful.

These four principles can provide a guideline in psychotherapeutic practice to distinguish adaptive from less adaptive modes of response. Psychotherapy should serve to develop *flexible, context-sensitive* responses (reactions) to demands the client is confronted with and to anchor these coping responses in the life of the person concerned (*retention*). Clients are assisted in therapy to select and apply those modes of response that will help them achieve their goals. These goals are based on a client's personal values and lead to an increase in psychological stability. Not only are the effects of the therapy process considered for the individual but also the interpersonal effects.

The following example of a client with anorexia nervosa will be used to describe how the evolution model helps to assess the maladaptivity of anorexic behavior at different system levels. As an aid to this procedure, Worksheet 14 (Assessment of Adaptivity) can be used. The matrix allows the therapist to assess the four evolutionary principles on each relevant system dimension and at a physiological and a sociocultural level (see Figure 51). In some cases, the influence of one dimension or system level is enough to limited adaptivity. For example, strong cognitive fusion alone may reduce variation, selection, retention, and context sensitivity substantially and prevent behaving adaptively. Therapy would target cognitive fusion, aiming at enhancing defusion. If therapy succeeds, this should lead to an increase in flexibility, adapted to the context and one's goals.

In Case Study 3.1, all dimensions of an anorexic client are strongly affected and contribute to the fact that strong and persistent restrictive eating is rarely adaptive.

Case Study 3.1. Amelie, client with anorexia nervosa

On an *emotional level*, Amelie, the anorexic client described in Figure 51, shows low competencies and little flexibility in handling her feelings. Amelie has difficulties differentiating feelings and to interpret or process emotional information. Instead of feeling "sad" or "disappointed," she often just feels "bad" and wants to feel "good." In addition, she has no idea how to react to different feelings or difficulties. Mostly, she just tries to avoid or hide negative feelings. When asked what else she could do, she has no repertoire to draw from. So mostly she focuses on "pulling herself together," trying to stay in control and at least try to appear happy. Unfortunately, smiling away problems does not solve them but causes more and more problems to arise, so that the energy expended on maintaining relative equilibrium steadily increases.

On a *cognitive level* she is strongly absorbed and fused with thoughts concerning her appearance, weight, or eating. The thought: "being thin and keeping control of myself makes me feel self-confident" persists, even though she experiences a steady deterioration of self-esteem in line with her loss of weight.

With regard to *attention*, equally noticeable is her narrow and rigid focus on details. She gets stuck on details (e.g., weighing 49.8 kg is tolerable, while exceeding 50 kg is intolerable and initiates suicidal thoughts), when distancing from the mere number on the scale and taking the broader focus on wanting to regain strength and energy would be helpful. Her attentional focus is narrowed to avoidance processes, such as "don't gain weight," "never weigh more than 50 kg," or "don't feel sad." Although harmful, she is not able to zoom out to see the bigger picture necessary to enable flexibility.

In relation to the *"self,"* she appears empty and passive ("nobody home phenomena"). The client does not resonate in situations and hardly connects with others. The "self" appears one-dimensional, it is largely defined by her occupation with her figure and weight and shows little context sensitivity.

> Her *behavior* is in accordance with the previously described rigidity, narrowed, ritualized, and avoidant, focused on maintaining control and preventing weight gain. She is unable to give up control to engage in experimental learning, like trying something new and evaluating its outcome.
>
> *Motivation* is dominated by avoidance goals, which override most other motivational processes.
>
> On the *physiological level*, the client shows deficiency symptoms as a result of malnutrition, such as lack of strength, and somatic sequelae.
>
> On the *social level*, the client does not seem connected to others. She has a limited perception of social processes. She cannot accept social support and is socially insecure.

Not all system dimensions or levels need to always play a maintaining role of a maladaptive network, as is the described case of a client with an eating disorder. With the help of the evolutionary matrix (Worksheet 14), it is possible to find out whether a particular dimension or level of processing is responsible for the network being dysfunctional, i.e., consuming a lot of energy even though it is not adapted to the problem and context. Case Study 3.2, describing a depressed client (see Hayes, Hofmann, & Ciarrochi, 2020), shows that although all system levels or dimensions are affected by the depression, the affective and cognitive levels are mainly responsible for the reduced adaptivity (see Figure 52). The affected person rigidly sticks to one strategy (rumination) and avoids experiencing emotions. This strategy is used globally and is therefore not context sensitive; moreover, it requires constant energy.

Worksheet 14

Evaluating Adaptivity Through the Extended Evolutionary Metamodel (Hayes & Hofmann, 2020)

		Variation	Selection	Retention	Context
Dimensions	Emotion	Avoiding emotions as main strategy	False display: no flexible repertoire	Pretending all is fine consumes more and more energy	Generalized strategy of playing a role pretending all is fine is not sensitive to the context
	Cognition	Fusion with inflexible eating-disorder-specific cognitions	Overgeneralizing of disorder-specific cognitions leads to rigid selection	Being constantly absorbed by weight-related thoughts costs energy	Overgeneralizing cognitions focused on weight and body are little context sensitive
	Attention	Inflexible toward threatening stimuli	–	Focus: Avoidance	–
	Self	Rigid, 1–dimensional, "nobody home"	Self-focused and defined by weight and body	–	Self disconnected from context
	Overt behavior	Little variation, rigid rituals	Oriented toward avoidance goals	Eating disorder behavior overrides other behaviors	–
	Motivation	Reduced to avoiding weight gain and creating control	–	Avoidance costs permanent energy	Disconnected from contextual influences
Levels	Biophysiological	Disturbed self-regulation	Self-harming strategies	Energy consuming strategy to prevent set-point regulation	Malnutrition reduces context sensitivity
	Sociocultural	Reduced interaction on a social level	Self-isolating and distancing from social connections	–	Disconnected from social context

Figure 51. Example of behavioral adaptivity assessment: Amelie, a client with anorexia nervosa. Blank version avalablie in Worksheet 14.

148   **Chapter 9**

Case Study 3.2. Steve, a depressed client

Steve, a depressed client, is very caught up in his brooding thoughts and fused with his thinking, he describes as a tight spiral of negative thoughts. Asked about his feelings, he reports emotional numbness. He feels empty and is absorbed by his negative thoughts. His attention revolves around these thoughts, and he confuses his thinking with his self. He believes he is inferior because of the way he thinks about himself and the more he thinks about it, the more hopeless he gets. This vicious circle produces depressive symptoms and disconnects him from others and his environment.

Worksheet 14

Evaluating Adaptivity Through the Extended Evolutionary Metamodel

		Variation	Selection	Retention	Context
Dimensions	Emotion	Avoidance, suppression	Strategy doesn't work	Needs permanent energy	Too unspecific
	Cognition	Fusion with thoughts	Worsens problem	Needs constant energy	Unspecific
	Attention	Rigid toward dysf. thoughts	–	–	Disconnected from context
	Self	Fusion with neg. self	Narrowed and rigid self offers less variability for selection	–	–
	Overt behavior	Avoidant	Enhances problem	Needs constant energy	unspecific
	Motivation	Avoidance goals	–	Avoidance requires permanent energy	unspecific
Levels	Biophysiological	High tension	Automatic responses reduce variability and selection	–	unspecific
	Sociocultural	Withdrawn	–	Loneliness is energy consuming	–

Figure 52.   Example of behavioral adaptivity assessment: Steve, a client with depression. Blank version avalablie in Worksheet 14.

9.3   Practical Example

To illustrate the work with the process-based complex network model, we will present a further, more complex case in which the network model formed the basis of a dynamic, transdiagnostic intervention model (see Case Study 3.3).

Case Study 3.3. Julia, a client with PTSD and depression

Initial situation. Julia is a 19-year-old kindergarten teacher who was raped two years earlier by her uncle during a camping trip. This traumatic experience, concealed from her family, triggered typical PTSD symptoms: intrusions, hyperarousal, intense feelings of shame, disgust, and fear, nightmares, and sleep disturbances. Overwhelmed by her feelings and thoughts, she tried to avoid triggering situations, proximity and contact with her family and other people, memories, and the emergence of unpleasant feelings.

Process-based diathesis model. The findings from the detailed diagnostic process were first summarized in a process-based diathesis model. In this model, the rape was selected as the external trigger, which leads to numerous internal challenges and psychological overloads, e.g., dealing with intense feelings of shame, disgust, guilt, and fear. Furthermore, Julia was overwhelmed with the intrusive images and the continuous emotional tension, as well as with the interpersonal challenge of carrying such a secret and not knowing how to deal with family situations involving the uncle. As a central vulnerability, very negative self-schemas already existed before the event, with the basic assumption of being worthless and a pronounced self-uncertainty associated with it. Predominant response mechanism was avoidance: physically, emotionally, and mentally. At work and with family and friends she tried as best she could to suppress or endure disturbing memories, images, and unpleasant feelings and avoid unpleasant or anxiety-provoking situations. When her feelings got unbearable, she resorted to the use of alcohol, hitting herself, and excessive exercise as coping strategies, hoping the "horror would go away." Entangled in these unpleasant states, trying to escape her own thoughts and feelings, it did not take long until she developed further depressive symptoms.

9.3.1 Individual Process-Based Complex Network Model

At first glance, the complex network model developed on the basis of these identified core processes (see Figure 53) looks complicated. However, it represents the actual complexity of the disorder and at the same time it integrates and reduces the comorbid disorders to a few relevant processes pulled together in one overall model. Firstly, the typical effects of the sexual assault are captured in the light gray boxes: intrusions, hyperarousal, and intense feelings. The model also indicates typical coping attempts (white), which aim at avoiding or suppressing these unpleasant symptoms. Thus, these coping attempts backfire and exacerbate PTSD symptoms (curved block arrows) and additionally contribute to the development of depressive symptoms via social withdrawal. The preexisting negative self-schema was identified as an important vulnerability for both disorder domains (hexagon). This vulnerability made it particularly difficult for Julia to deal with what she had experienced and to initiate active coping behaviors, such as seeking help. At the same time, the activated negative-self scheme intensified other depressive processes. The depressive symptoms revolved around the following dimensions: negative affect, withdrawal, and negative thinking about herself and the world.

9.3.2 Complexity

At this point, as a therapist, one should not be afraid of complexity. What Julia experienced was actually much more complex than the model shown in Figure 53 can reflect. The client experienced this model as a simplification because it neglects many stressful details that are not relevant to the disorder dynamics. At the same time, it includes indi-

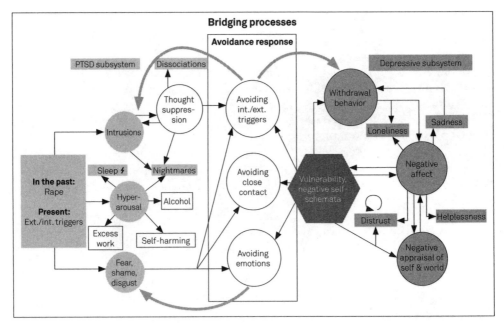

Figure 53. Complex network model of Julia (PTSD and major depression).

vidual aspects, such as self-injury, alcohol abuse, isolation, or interactional problems in relationships, without assigning them a disease value of their own. Looking at the model, it all made sense to her and became less "crazy." On a categorial level of *DSM* or *ICD*, she may have been diagnosed not only with a PTSD, but also an alcohol problem, presumably an emotional instability with self-harm tendencies. By integrating the reactions into a superordinate model, they are given a logic in the overall context.

9.3.3 Core Dimensions

By repeatedly discussing situations and placing them in the network model, it was possible to limit the treatment focus to two essential core dimensions: global avoidance and negative self-concept. These two reinforcing dimensions limited Julia's coping attempts and contributed to the increasing elaboration of the trauma network, making her increasingly depressed. Julia could easily perceive the maladaptiveness of her coping with trauma because she herself experienced it as confining, rigid, and energy consuming.

9.3.4 Accessing Adaptivity

Using the matrix for assessing adaptivity, Julia recognized the ineffective rigidity of her attempts to cope. "At the moment I survive from day to day, but I'm not going anywhere in my broken life," she would put it. The problem was, she did not know any alternative ways of reacting except to flee from unpleasant situations and feelings (little variation and selection). She expressed that it cost her more and more strength to endure life (missing retention), and this would override all situations in life (context).

10
Phase 4: Defining Therapy Goals and Creating Readiness for Change

10.1 Defining Global Therapy Goals

As at the beginning of any therapy, the global therapy goals must be defined. Where is the joint journey going? What do we want to achieve at the end? Many clients want to "feel better," or assume by going to therapy that disturbing psychological symptoms like sleeplessness or anxiety will automatically disappear. These nonspecific wishes are usually only the starting point for defining concrete therapy goals. Wanting something to go away is not the same as wanting to overcome the forces of an entrenched network. Therefore, from a process-based perspective, the development of a desirable vision (attractor state) in the sense of "What will your life be like if therapy is successful?" is essential. "What do you want to actually achieve through therapy?" is important as an overarching approach goal. This goal serves both as a compass for the desired change and as an attractor state that can help build up a stable pull motivation for the change process. A depressed client might express that she wants to participate in life again, connect socially, and pursue her interests more actively. A client with anorexia nervosa may desire to regain the strength to focus finishing school or university, be open to a relationship, and have the confidence to decide if she wants a family. It is important that these goals not be general phrases but are personally important goals connected to individual motives and values. The client must *convince* the therapist that the new state is a truly important concern to her. In the following sections we will stick to describing the process-based steps in the treatment of Julia, the young client suffering from PTSD and depression. First, we will look at how therapy goals were defined.

Case Study 3.4. Julia, the described client with PTSD and depression

Julia, like many clients, initially *only* wanted "the terrible symptoms to go away." She wanted to get rid of the images, memories, and nightmares. Also "the tension should disappear," because otherwise she would "go crazy." Therefore, the time frame was extended to a medium-term future, with the question, "How do you want to look back on the events a year from now, when you have managed to cope with them better? What is worth taking on a stressful trauma therapy?" Julia was then able to gradually formulate global goals:

1. "I don't want this event to destroy my life. I want to survive it."
2. "I want to move on with my life. Study, have friends, find trust in people again."
3. "I want to be able to look my family and friends in the eye again."
4. Later, in the course of therapy, she added, "I want to be able to accept myself and my life as it is."

10.2 Defining Targets of Change at a Process Level

Based on the global therapy goals, the next question, when looking at the complex network model, is: "Which of these process-level mechanisms need to change specifically to achieve the higher-level therapy goals?" If the client is stuck in this network of intertwining processes, which process needs to change to get unstuck? Where do I apply the crowbar to obtain the most leverage for the client to overcome the forces of a pathological network dominating their life? (see Case Study 3.5).

Case Study 3.5. Julia, the client with PTSD and depression

In Julia's case, it was possible to use the complex network model to find numerous starting points to disrupt the current pathological dynamic and to initiate change. She was able to look at the model from a metaperspective, make her own reflections, and suggest goals, such as: "If only I didn't always blame myself for everything" or "if these feelings wouldn't just crush me" or "If I could muster the courage to talk to my parents" or "If I could talk about what happened without breaking down." From this distance, she was able to see solutions, she just lacked the faith that she could find the courage to face her fears. From this, concrete process goals could gradually be defined:

1. *Reduction of avoidance* on the mental, behavioral, and emotional level while simultaneously developing competencies in dealing with unpleasant feelings and thoughts. This should weaken the reinforcing feedbacks (see the curved arrows in Figure 52) to the PTSD symptoms.
2. *Learning to deal with high tension* (instead of dissociation, alcohol, self-harm). Already during the formulation of point 1, Julia got into a strongly pronounced high tension and was thus able to express the wish that she wanted to improve the way she dealt with it.
3. *Exposure-oriented trauma processing* that addresses PTSD symptoms. Julia realized that she could not spend a lifetime "keeping a lid on what had happened." She recognized herself in a PTSD metaphor in which trying to suppress thoughts and feelings is similar to standing in a lake trying to push air-filled balls under the surface so that nobody notices them, while at the same time trying to act relaxed and normal. It is impossible to pay attention all the time to prevent the memories and feelings from surfacing and life becomes very dull and stressful when both hands are consumed with keeping thoughts and feelings away. She understood that she will have to let go and let the thoughts and feelings surface if she wants to be freed from being permanently attached to the traumatic events. She could fully understand the confrontation rationale.
4. *Modification of the negative self-schema:* During the diagnostic phase, Julia developed an awareness of her devastating self-deprecations. She was downright shocked at how aggressively and negatively she mentally treated herself. She was so focused on aggressively blaming herself (e.g., for the experienced sexual assault) and thinking negatively about herself, she didn't think of directing this aggression against the perpetrator. Reducing the negative thought spirals and learning to stand by herself and take care of herself were important learning goals in therapy. It took time for Julia to see her own way of dealing

with herself as a limiting factor for coping. It helped her to ask herself how she would help a child from her kindergarten who confided in her. Would she shower it with accusations and recommend: "Keep it to yourself and try to forget it. It's probably your fault!" With this perspective, Julia was able to formulate more self-compassionate and helpful ways she would help another person and these ideas were of course helpful for her own healing process.

5. *Learning to discriminate between anxiety and danger* in order to interrupt automated avoidance responses. In the course of time her anxiety had generalized to many situations, including closeness to others, experiencing feeling involving uncertainty and being open. In this way, her conditioned anxiety was associated with her viewing many day-to-day situations as dangerous. Learning to discriminate between her anxiety and the evaluation of a situation as dangerous or safe aimed at weakening "global avoidance" and increasing context sensitivity.

6. *Establishing connection and trust with self* (compassion) and others (trust) to change negative self-concept.

10.3 Capturing Readiness for Change

Even if the starting points for change in therapy are obvious, a stable motivation for change is required throughout the course of therapy in order to overcome the pathological network state. For example, a client with anorexia nervosa may desire nothing more than to eat normally and regain strength and energy, but treatment will activate fears of gaining weight and require constant motivation for change for several years. If she is not able to keep up the required motivation to resist falling back into typical eating-disorder behaviors, progress once made will quickly deteriorate, which leads to further demoralization. The desire to get well is therefore not enough to sustain a continuous change response.

10.3.1 Determining the Current Phase of Motivation

As already explained in Section 4.3.4, the motivation to change requires five transformation steps, which are continuously guided by therapy (see also Figure 33 on p. 86): The client must first *recognize* their own problems and resistances and *decide to* behave contrary to previous patterns. This decision must be *implemented in* concrete terms. This means overcoming oneself again and again, acting contrary to automated reactions and *maintaining* the change. A client goes through this cycle in every therapy sequence.

In this constantly flowing process, it is not very helpful to say that a client "is or is not motivated." Rather, it must be specified in which phase of motivation the client is and to which dimension of change the state of motivation refers. Motivation represents a core process of change – a mediator variable in relation to all processes that are to be changed – and should therefore be considered at every point in the therapy. In addition, the current phase of motivation may differ for different subprocesses. For example, a client with an eating disorder may formulate a *desire for* "self-esteem enhancement" (wish) and *de-*

154   Chapter 10

cide to work on the body schema disorder (implementation), but she may *not yet recognize a* need for change with respect to adequate food intake (*denial*). In order to be able to determine the current position in the motivation cycle, it is helpful to look at and discuss it together with the client. The first page of Worksheet 15 (Motivation for Change; see Appendix) can be used for this purpose.

Since motivation to change is a central process for therapy, it is recommended to explicitly discuss the factors that are prerequisites for a firm decision for change. Willingness to change is determined by the costs and benefits (valence), the importance (salience) of a change in relation to the status quo, and the assessment of the likelihood of achieving the therapy goal (Berking & Kowalsky, 2012). The second page of Worksheet 15 contains corresponding questions that the clients can clarify for themselves.

For the therapy process, motivation to change is a core process. The success or failure of a therapy is often determined by whether the client can be gently guided from one motivation phase to the next. If this is not the case, it is the therapist's task to make this transparent and to select therapeutic interventions aimed at promoting the motivational process. According to the motivation model of Prochaska and DiClemente (1983), at this point it is often a matter of moving from the state of passive "wanting" (treatment motivation) to an action-oriented "resolution" (change motivation).

There are cases in which clients deny their problems and externalize them exclusively, looking for an ally in the therapist. Or, clients recognize their problems and think that this insight is already enough to change something. These clients do not get beyond the wishing stage. They may have recognized that something is going wrong and ardently wish for a change, such as more self-worth, less anxiety, or less misery, but do not derive from this a purposeful resolution to take certain actions that must precede any change process.

10.3.2 Cost-Benefit Analysis for Change

The client should be able to convince you, the therapist, that (1) they understand that wishing alone will not bring about change, and (2) they can realistically estimate the benefits and costs of change. Further, the client should (3) be able to convince you why the change is so important to them personally (salience), and (4) anticipate that they have the capability to succeed (positive outcome prognosis).

Statements like "It would be nice if I could be more cheerful again" are not convincing. I (M. S.) react to this with provocative interventions by saying: "Oh, cheerfulness is overrated. After all, you are now used to being depressed and hardly know yourself any different. I think you should stick with that concept of depression. Or can you give me a *real* reason to go through the trouble of therapy?" This emphasizes that change does not just happen but requires willingness, overcoming, and perseverance. The resistance built up by such a paradoxical intervention is small compared to the resistance the person must overcome in therapy. It is not uncommon for clients to respond to such a provocation something like, "Yeah, maybe you're right. That's what I always tell myself, and nothing will change anyway." It then makes no sense to ignore this deep negative belief and continue with the interventions that are bound to fail.

Instead, clarifying the components of the required motivation through a cost-benefit analysis helps the client build up the goal-oriented motivation that is needed to overcome a pathological network state and establish a new coping network. Worksheet 16 (Cost-Bene-

Table 7. Cost-benefit analysis for treatment

	Advantages/benefits	Disadvantages/costs
Previous handling of the challenges	• What desired effect is achieved by the current handling? • What negative effects are currently being prevented? • What other benefits does the status quo have?	• What does this also prevent? What will I miss out on as a result? • What are the downsides of the status quo in the long run? • What are the side effects of currently dealing with my problems?
Dealing with the challenges through therapy	• What benefits are hoped for? • What would be the overall impact of a change? • What is worth fully engaging in therapy for?	• What disadvantages do I fear? • What problems does this create? • What am I afraid might happen if I pull through and change? • What do I have to do to deal with then?

Case Study 3.6. Julia, a client with PTSD and depression

Julia was initially in the "wishing" phase in which she hoped her unpleasant memories, permanent arousal and avoidance would just disappear. The resolution to confront herself actively with her unpleasant internal and external states had not yet matured. When discussing realistic goals, she became aware of the costs holding her back: "I can never tell my father what happened" or "I can't bear the memories. I will just go crazy and end up in a psychiatric ward." Discussing and analyzing the motivational phases of change, Julia was able to localize herself in the "wishing" stage, so we first dealt with the development of a "resolution to change" before beginning actual interventions targeting PTSD symptoms. For this, she intensively examined the costs, benefits, and importance of achieving her global goals (cost-benefit analysis).

fit Analysis for Treatment in the Appendix) can be used for this purpose. The questions help elicit (see also Table 7) significant benefits for the client, but also the costs of changing. In this way, the client can examine whether the motivation to change is sufficient to tolerate the expected negative consequences (costs) and thus to be able to achieve their long-term goal. Such a cost-benefit analysis can help to strengthen the decision-making process with regard to the desired change through treatment (therapy) and thus generate motivation to change (see Case Study 3.6).

10.3.3 Determining the Type and Duration of Motivation Required for Change

To illustrate the importance of developing the right kind of motivation to the kind of change process I am engaged with, we will look at everyday challenges. It makes a big difference if I am motivating myself for a one-time action or if I have to make a resolution for a change I have to keep up for many years. For example, I might be carrying around the idea of exchanging a lamp in the attic for some time, talking about it every now and then for some years. Here I have spent years in the "wishing phase" until I make the resolution to change something and get engaged in the necessary activity. In this example the difficult thing is to get out of the precontemplation phase and make a decision for a one-time action. You have to give yourself a push, but if you cross the threshold that's holding you back, then you're quickly in the implementation phase. It's like bracing to ride up a short steep hill with a bicycle. Once you have got started, you have nearly done it.

Not all desired changes require this short decisive motivational kick start. If I resolve to learn to play the guitar or learn a language, this method doesn't work. While the first example requires a short period of focused high motivation, the second situation requires maintaining the stable motivation to change over a long period of time. This is like the difference between a sprint and a marathon. Some changes, like learning to play an instrument, require taking lessons and practicing regularly for years. In therapy, we are often confronted with different kinds of changes, for which we have to establish the right kind of motivation. Some therapy goals need a short phase of decisive, strong, and focused motivation to overcome a high threshold holding someone back. Other goals require a completely different

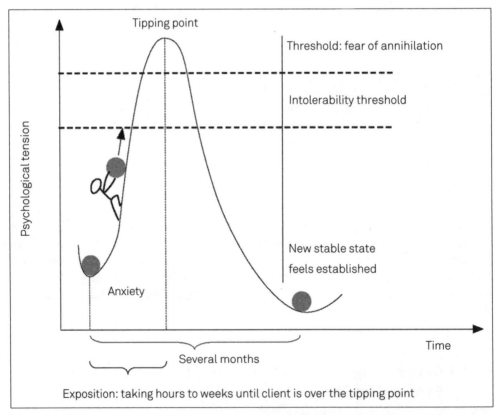

Figure 54. Schematic course of change in an anxiety treatment. Exposure treatment requires a brief but very strong willingness to change with a firm commitment to a specific intervention. This requires a confrontation with subjectively intolerable, sometimes annihilating feelings, until the client settles in a new stable state.

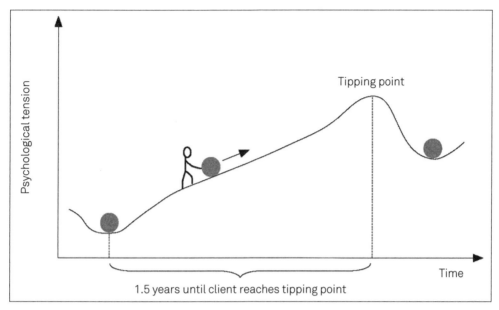

Figure 55. Schematic process of changing dysfunctional self-schemas by means of self-verbalization techniques. The process of change leading to the tipping point takes place over a very long period of time and requires a continuous flow of motivational energy – sometimes for months to years.

kind of motivation in which the client has to keep up a constant dose of motivation for a long-term change process. Figures 54 to 56 illustrate the change process using the mountain-and-valley model and use this visualization to clarify the different demands on the motivation process.

Figure 54 shows the course of an anxiety treatment using exposure therapy. One can see a steeply progressing but temporally short phase of change. The motivation driving the client to confront themselves must be high for the short period in which the exposures take place and sufficiently enable the client to remain in the exposure situations. We can prepare our client, developing a willingness to engage in the therapeutic rationale of exposure by predicting what they will experience in this confrontation phase and how their reaction will develop: "your arousal will rise to a maximum, until you will notice a slow decline after 30 to 60 minutes." The closer our predictions reflect the client's experience, the more likely they will have faith in the therapy rationale and stay in the confronting situation.

The situation is different when the core process to be changed is a rigid, negative schema, like the belief of being an unworthy person. The motivation required to use an affirmation technique to modify a schema must be more consistent and long-lasting than that required for an exposure treatment (see Figure 55) – comparable to the motivation required to learn an instrument. A strong will to change is not enough. Change happens slowly and over a long period of time. The motivation to change must therefore be secured through structures and habits, otherwise the individual will run out of steam by the tipping point at which the change is anchored. From a network perspective, change occurs through repeatedly and gradually changing network links until the old links have been sufficiently weakened and the helpful beliefs have been anchored to create a more favorable network.

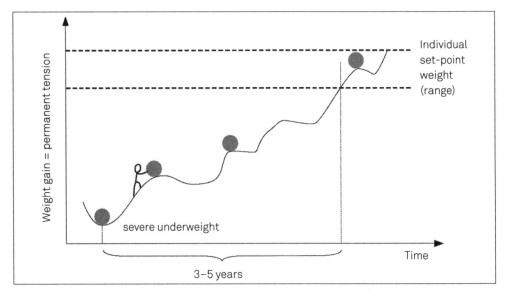

Figure 56. Schematic weight development in the treatment of anorexia nervosa. To increase and stabilize weight, a long-lasting motivation to change is required for coping processes over a period of years. Motivation problems can arise due to the duration of therapy as well as the psychological tension that increases with weight. The tension is reduced only after the set-point.

Finally, Figure 56 shows the weight gain in the treatment of anorexia nervosa, visualizing the disruption of an eating disorder network over the course of treatment and the development of a healthier coping network. The coping process will realistically take years, requiring the client to apply coping techniques on a daily basis for a very long period of time (e.g., using eating protocols and focusing on fixed meal structure). Willpower or a one-time willingness to change are not sufficient to fuel an ongoing change process in which there is no quick relief. On the contrary, staying motivated gets more difficult, the more weight is gained. Even when the client has reached her individual set-point weight, eating-disorder symptoms, typically disturbing thoughts and body sensations, will permanently trigger the impulse to reduce weight. The "set-point" is the individual weight range of a person with regular and sufficient nutrition; in this biologically set range, which is healthy for the individual, self-regulatory eating based on hunger and satiety sets in. In the treatment of anorexia, however, the weight phobia initially becomes stronger as weight increases, and at the same time the suffering caused by being underweight decreases. The risk of discontinuation increases as therapy becomes more successful because it becomes more difficult to maintain a motivation to change. The terraced progression in Figure 56 depicts an interval-based therapeutic approach and at the same time reflects the gradual remodeling of the eating-disorder network. This remodeling occurs in stages in which the affected person repeatedly reaches plateaus on which the new structure can stabilize before striving for a new target state that requires renewed destabilization. For each stage, the specific motivation for change must be built up again, and the clients must be prepared for the fact that relief will not come very soon, as is the case with other change processes. Psychological relief is not to be expected until the client's weight has settled for a longer period of time within the set-point range.

10.3.4 Subjective Prognosis of Success Limits Change

Finally, the subjective prognosis of goal achievement is a decisive factor in enabling an individual to make a decision to change. To do this, the client needs to know what kind of change they are signing up for. Is the resolution for a short exposure or a one-event change or is it a resolution for a change that requires a long-term commitment as in the case of many therapeutic goals that involve a constant change of behavior or thinking?

Even if the decision to change has been made, assessing the expectation of success is important in order to actually take action. Illustrated with an example: When running up to jump over a brook I will constantly evaluate if I will make the distance. If the answer to this constant evaluation is "No, I'll probably end up in the water," I will abandon the attempt beforehand. Sticking with the "jumping over the stream" picture, one would probably only jump when the probability of success is very high (e.g., over 85%). In therapy, clients are constantly engaged in assessing if therapy will successfully help to resolve their problems. As soon as their assessment of success dips, motivation for change is scrapped and therapy comes to a halt. The scale shown in Box 12 can be used for prognosis assessment by both the client *and* the therapist (see also Worksheet 15, on which the prognosis can be assessed by the client and the therapist).

Box 12. Forecast assessment

> Do you think you will achieve the therapy goals with the proposed method? How high do you estimate the probability (0 to 100%)?
>
> 0% —— 25% —— 50% —— 75% —— 100%
>
> This aspect of clients permanently calculating costs and benefits and their subjective success expectation as a moderator for change motivation is sometimes overlooked. If the cost-benefit calculation clearly speaks in favor of a change, but the affected person does not expect to succeed (low success probability), they will not actively engage in the proposed change process, or at least hesitate. This is often the case with pronounced demoralization after many failed attempts to change (see Case Study 3.7 Julia, client with PTSD and depression).

Case Study 3.7. Julia, client with PTSD and depression

> Taking Julia's negative self-schemas into account, she was subjectively very pessimistic that she could change the situation she felt stuck in. She had read that one always remains "mentally broken" after a trauma. Objectively, Julia had many resources (intelligence, relational strength, family support), and she demonstrated a good understanding of the therapy rationale. Thus, the problem was not a lack of skills but a lack of confidence in herself and low self-esteem limiting her change motivation. To make sure Julia had the necessary motivation, she was asked to estimate her success probability. While she noticed that at the beginning of therapy she had not really believed that it would be possible to change anything (success rate <15%), she was already more optimistic and gave herself a 65% success probability after the first few sessions. After assessing her deficits and resources, the therapist saw the success probability by at least 85%. By discussing the discrepancy, it was still

possible to discuss Julia's worries and open questions and to correct some of Julia's misconceptions, so that at the end of the sessions analyzing her commitment and motivation she increased her success estimate to 80 %.

This is the most favorable case in which both client and therapist can realistically believe in a positive outcome. But what do you do, when the client sees little hope in creating a difference and this bleak perspective is shared from a therapeutic standpoint? Sometimes reality sucks, but it doesn't make sense to negate reality. If there is little chance of success, it is important to revise the therapy goals, redefining goals the client can reach with the help of psychotherapy. In the case of a chronic depressive client who united many risk factors and had a long history of suicide attempts, he realized that the wish "to get rid of the depression and lead a happy life" was not realistic. This hope had in the past led to disappointments and frustration, causing him to abandon previous therapies. A realistic goal to which he could commit himself was to prevent further deterioration, improve his management of depressive symptoms and crisis, establish a support network, and stay alive despite suffering from severe depression.

11
Phase 5: Selecting and Implementing Interventions

11.1 Selecting Interventions

Once the relevant core processes for the maintenance of the maladaptive dynamics on a process level have been identified and targeted changes defined by developing an individual, complex network model, interventions can be selected and implemented. Starting points for these interventions are central reaction mechanisms responsible for maintaining the maladaptive network.

11.1.1 Defining Effective Dimensions to Target

At this point, in process-based therapy, it is important to define the desired effect of therapy based on the individual network model: What effect does one want to achieve in order to change the network? If one has created an individual network model in which the fusion with dysfunctional thoughts (e.g., "Others reject me") is highly responsible for the spread of depressiogenic patterns (e.g., withdrawal, avoidance behavior, loss of self-esteem), one will define the defusion from these thoughts as a dimension to target. This decision is based on the hypothesis that weakening the fusion with this core belief should have a beneficial effect on the other depressive symptoms. Defusion with this belief should lead to a noticeable reduction of avoidance behavior, withdrawal, and an improvement in self-esteem. Once therapist and client agree that the desired changes require the client's distancing themselves from this negative core belief, possible interventions can be discussed. This could include practicing defusion strategies or using reattribution and self-verbalization techniques. Having consensus between the therapist and the client on the therapy rationale is crucial for the success of the interventions. If the client does not understand the mechanism of action (e.g., specific fusion causes depression) or does not believe in the effect of defusion, the implementation of interventions is not promising.

Table 8 summarizes the evidence-based impact factors identified by Kazantzis and colleagues (2018) in a comprehensive review of meta-analyses. In principle, these are a manageable number of therapeutic strategies that therapists need to translate into personalized interventions. This compilation can also be found on Worksheet 17 (see Appendix).

Table 8. Evidence-based impact factors in psychotherapy (based on Kazantzis et al., 2018)

System level	Impact factors
Therapy process (change process)	
Cognitive processes	• Decentering (e.g., defusion, mindfulness, detached mindfulness) • Attention focus
Cognitions	• Reevaluation • Reframing • Increase self-efficacy expectation • Modify outcome expectation
Behavior	• Confrontation • Behavioral activation
Emotion regulation	• Acceptance
Motivation	• Clarity regarding therapy goals • Values
Session process (therapeutic interaction)	
—	• Therapeutic relationship (alliance) • Consensus on therapy goals and collaboration • Feedback on the course of therapy • Homework

11.1.2 Selecting Interventions to Change Core Processes

There are a number of established and empirically validated therapeutic methods and procedures that therapists can resort to in order to change the core processes listed in Chapter 4. The standard methods named by the Inter-Organizational Task Force on Cognitive and Behavioral Psychology Doctoral Education (Klepac et al., 2012) are assigned to the core processes of psychopathology or the corresponding system levels at which they are located in Table 9 (the table can also be found on Worksheet 18; see Appendix). The purpose of this comparison is to illustrate that the empirically well-validated methods for process-based psychotherapy do not need to be reinvented. Rather, the Task Force's summary confirms that the interventions applied and found to be important in successful therapies are those that address the core processes of psychopathology.

The implementation of interventions in the process-based approach does not differ from the CBT standard procedures. Essential for process-based therapy is linking interventions to individual core processes that are responsible for maintaining a maladaptive condition within a process-based complex model.

Whether a problematic process is relevant to the maintaining dynamics of the disorder can only be decided on a case-by-case basis. For example, in many cases avoidance behavior may be maladaptive and central to the maintenance of a disorder. Avoidance hinders reevaluating a situation, habituation, and the development of self-efficacy. But this does not mean that avoidance is per se a problematic reaction. Many people avoid difficult situations in life without the avoidance behavior becoming generalized or contributing to (further) psychological symptoms. In these cases, avoidance just makes life easier and is not in my therapeutic focus. Only if the avoidance behavior gets out of hand, generalizes, or elicits problematic emotional or cognitive processes are we dealing with a relevant psychopathological core process.

In summary, under a process-based perspective, the selection of interventions is guided by (1) the impact of the process for the maintenance of psychopathology and (2) whether it serves the purpose of achieving the client's global therapeutic goal (see Case Study 3.8).

Table 9. Standard psychotherapeutic procedures for targeted interventions (based on Klepac et al., 2012) for core processes of psychopathology (see also Hofmann & Hayes, 2018)

Core processes of psychopathology (according to system level)	Standard psychotherapeutic procedures
Somatic regulation processes	• Tension reduction
Behavioral processes	• Contingency management • Stimulus Control • Shaping • Self-management • Exposure therapies • Behavior building and activation • Behavioral training
Emotion regulation processes	• Coping and emotion regulation (also exposure) • Acceptance
Cognitive processes	• Problem-solving therapy • Attentional training • Cognitive reappraisal • Modification of core beliefs • Defusion • Value clarification
Social and interpersonal processes	• Interpersonal skills training
Multidimensional constructs	• Mindfulness training • Enhancing motivation • Crisis management and suicidality management

Case Study 3.8. Julia, client with PTSD and depression

In the case of Julia – the young, traumatized woman – the interventions listed in Box 13 below were selected for the process goals formulated in therapy.

164　Chapter 11

Box 13. Linking process objectives to concrete interventions

Process targets and concrete interventions

Dealing with heightened arousal and emotional tension levels
- Learning to deal with high tension (rather than dissociation, alcohol, self-harm) by monitoring tension and using tension regulation techniques (e.g., anchoring techniques, breathing techniques, defusion techniques)
- Learning to recognize and end dissociations

Reducing avoidance behavior
- Creating awareness for avoidance behaviors through self-observation sheets
- Understanding the role of avoidance and the exposure rationale
- Exposures

Dealing with trauma induced images and negative schemas
- Rescripting and reprocessing traumatic memories through imagery rescripting and reprocessing therapy (IRRT)

Modification of the negative self-schemas
- Weakening negative schemata through cognitive restructuring and defusion
- Strengthening the self in context and defusing from thoughts defining the traumatized self as "broken"
- Establishing connection and trust with self (compassion) and others (trust)
- Developing and practicing a self-compassion affirmation

Learning to direct the attention to help create safety
- Learning to distinguish between anxiety and danger
- Discrimination learning in relation to different triggers: men, closeness, familiarity, openness

11.1.3 Planning the Sequence of Interventions

At the beginning of the intervention phase, it can sometimes be difficult to decide what to begin with. Is it important to first minimize the effect of negative thoughts to lower the cognitive barriers to change, or does the client need concrete skills to cope with challenging emotional states? There is no universal answer to this question, but working with the complex network model helps to predict the effects of interventions, so very often the client can help make these decisions. In general, experiential and behavioral interventions (exposures, behavioral training) prove to be more effective than purely cognitive methods. It can be tempting to keep to the safe grounds of thinking about change and avoiding behavioral changes that might elicit strong emotional reactions. So, if therapy sessions feel too pleasant and lack emotional depth then maybe the client, the therapist, or both are avoiding core processes of change. Furthermore, the choice of interventions depends on the phase of therapy. In the initial phase of therapy, the focus is on interventions that help identify problems and build motivation (e.g., self-monitoring, cost-benefit analysis, goal clarification). Next, interventions that help the client to take a metalevel, i.e., to take a step back and develop an understanding of the problem, are useful. It only makes sense to select interventions that prompt change when there is high agreement regarding the understanding of the disorder and the rationale for therapy. In addition, motivational aspects, safety aspects, and practical considerations may influence the selection of interventions and thus require constant flexible adjustment of the therapeutic process to adapt the therapeutic strategy to the individual situation.

11.1.4 Weaken the Maladaptive Network or Strengthen the Coping Network?

From a network perspective, the change process in psychotherapy consists of weakening an established pathological network causing an individual to suffer while strengthening a more adaptive coping network. For example, a trauma network can be weakened by breaking automated links between trigger situations and intrusions, hyperarousal, and avoidance through confrontational interventions. These interventions destabilize the trauma network. The destabilized network enables the client to establish new adaptive linkages. In this newly established network, the client is anchored in the present moment, can detach from traumatic intrusions, and is able to apply self-soothing and tension-reducing techniques.

It seems important that the process of destabilizing the existing network and building an alternative network go hand in hand. It is of no use to destabilize a pathological network without working on an alternative. Conversely, it is not possible to build an alternative network without destabilizing the pathological network. From the network perspective, it is clear that the change process goes through a phase of instability. This is problematic in that, as a therapist, one has to explain to a client who is already at the breaking point that they must be prepared for greater instability. At this point, we would like to refer to Section 2.5, which uses Figure 15 to describe the gradual destabilization of the maladaptive network and the gradual building of an adaptive network.

11.2 Implementing Interventions

The essence of the process-based approach has already been explained. In the implementation phase of therapy, there is a scientifically based variety of methods based on the psychotherapeutic efficacy factors (Kazantzis et al., 2018) and the recognized standard procedures (Klepac et al., 2012). The specific means by which the implementation of interventions is achieved depends on the therapeutic training and experience of the therapists and on client variables. A therapist trained strictly in cognitive behavioral therapy (CBT) will prefer different interventions than a therapist trained in acceptance and commitment therapy (ACT). Many interventions have been developed in parallel in different theoretical contexts. As with different medications, it is not the "product name" that is essential, but the effect factor. As an example, distancing techniques, decentering methods, mindfulness-based techniques, defusion techniques, and detached-mindfulness techniques have a similar spectrum of effectiveness. Depending on the therapist's training or experience, the interventions with which one feels most confident are resorted to, so the selection follows theoretical and practical considerations. As long as the methodology is based on an individual process-based disease model and on the application of the recognized standard procedures, taking into account the scientifically justified effective factors, the individual approach to implementation is not a problem. Also, different client groups require different intervention approaches. For example, adolescents or cognitively impaired clients will require a more behavioral approach, making it more difficult to implement purely cognitive interventions.

12

Phase 6: Monitoring Change and Constant Reevaluation

Psychotherapy, as Persons (1989) describes, is an ongoing hypothesis-driven process of hypothesis generation, testing, and adjustment. An empirical process involves continuous progress monitoring, which allows the formulated hypotheses to be reevaluated. Monitoring progress in therapy leads to better therapeutic outcomes (Lambert, 2010). Additionally, it encourages active participation, increases clients' experience of efficacy and control, and reduces self-criticism (Antony et al., 2005).

The regulatory flexibility model already presented in Section 4.2.7 (Bonanno & Burton, 2013) describes quite well how psychotherapy focuses on helping individuals to adapt their reactions to challenging situations. This requires increasing regulatory flexibility by improving context sensitivity, i.e., concrete and realistic perception and evaluation of demands, and building skills and strategies (repertoire). The crucial component of the model leading to adaptive flexibility is the feedback loop constantly providing information on how good my attempts in finding the best coping response. Without a functioning feedback loop, there is no improvement in context sensitivity and no expansion of the repertoire.

It is not possible to get a process-based perturbation model "right" on the first try. Rather, it is a process that becomes more and more "right." Therefore, it always culminates in the analysis of the client's experience, the verification of the initially formulated hypotheses, and the verification of the effect by means of progress monitors. Are there deviations, and how can these be explained? What processes, if any, have been overlooked in the initial hypothesis? How does the perturbation model need to be supplemented? Which hypotheses result from this? What interventions would need to be adapted or supplemented?

To notice these deviations, it is important to measure the processes in focus and the effects on psychopathology. A wealth of disorder-specific test procedures exists for recording psychopathology. Regarding the recording of process variables, the methods of special process diagnostics presented in Section 7.10 can be used, other forms of symptom or progress diaries, or expert assessments that assess coping progress in certain domains of change. In principle, defining progress together with the client in the planning phase of therapy prevents therapy from getting lost in the woods. Leading questions for the discussion are:

- How do we know we are making progress in therapy?
- How can progress be measured and quantified?

12.1 Negative Versus Positively Oriented Monitors

In the diagnostic phase, problematic processes are often monitored to create awareness for these dimensions linked to the development of individual problems. The client may be asked to monitor how many hours a day they ruminate, spend in bed, spend at home or in their room, are inactive, or spend in disorder-related activities (e.g., vomiting, compulsions, PC gaming). Monitoring establishes a feedback loop connecting problematic processes to an outcome variable. "So, you spent 7 hours alone watching TV and your monitored mood deteriorated over that time span. What does that teach us?" This sets a baseline to experiment changing processes and watching what else changes, helping to identify starting points for change. So, at first the focus is on the problematic processes we want to change. Once we have identified these and we enter the treatment phase, it is advisable to repolarize the monitors so that the monitor is named after the desired target, thereby becoming an approach target. If, in the example of a depressed client spending most of the day alone, increasing social activity is a process goal, it makes sense to monitor not the number of hours spent alone but the number of hours the client spends time engaged with others. If one has identified inactivity as a problematic process in the diagnostic phase, in the intervention phase one would monitor the number of activities performed and the duration in which pleasurable activities are performed. In addition, it is more motivating to record, for example, the number of hours or days that a bulimic client does not vomit than to always record only when a relapse occurs.

12.2 Critical Thresholds and Bottlenecks in Therapy

The therapy process described is complex, and it is not always clear whether a stagnation in the progress of therapy represents a threshold phenomenon or means that no more can be achieved. In any treatment, there are always critical points or thresholds that are more difficult to overcome, such as facing shameful issues or confronting anxiety-provoking situations. In eating disorder therapy, this may be certain weight ranges; in obsessive-compulsive disorder, it may be giving up a certain safety behavior. Developments or learning processes are not linear: At times, one seems to be treading water, and then there are sudden improvements – so-called "sudden gains." Motivation is also subject to fluctuations, so that one day a client may confidently apply strategies and the next day no longer see any point in continuing therapy.

12.3 Criteria for Ending Therapy

Psychotherapy deals with developmental processes and adaptation processes. Basically, these never end, so it is sometimes difficult to define the point in time at which therapy should end. Sometimes the end of therapy is pushed further and further back, and new issues are found again and again. Or therapy becomes a self-perpetuating process because it undermines self-efficacy or autonomy. In some circumstances, therapy can become a habit that is resorted to for all problems. To avoid this, criteria for when the "work is done" should be defined early on. These criteria for ending therapy can best be noted when discussing therapy goals. The criteria should allow to define "ending therapy due to therapy success" and "ending therapy due to lack of progress."

13
Outlook

Klaus Grawe (Grawe & colleagues, 1994) already outlined the possibility of a process-based psychotherapy in the early 1990s and ventured a blueprint for a general psychotherapy. The background of this reflection was the long-lasting school controversy in psychotherapy, in which therapy methods and schools were tested against each other, rather than focusing on understanding the core processes of change. Klaus Grawe was convinced that psychotherapy, like other scientific disciplines, can only evolve by evaluating the mechanisms (processes) of psychopathology and effectors of change (Stangier, 2019).

Processes Instead of Methods

Although in the last 50 years the knowledge of evidence-based processes in psychopathology and the change process has grown substantially, diagnosis-oriented treatment manuals dominate clinical practice, and methods are applied nonspecifically to diagnostic categories in the hope that what works in general will work for the specific individual. Practicing therapists also prefer to read books on therapy procedures, treatment manuals, or therapy tools rather than on psychopathological mechanisms of action. Even the process-oriented third-wave methods, often developed as a counterpart to existing diagnosis-oriented approaches, threaten to develop into therapy schools and belief systems themselves. The typical opening conversation of psychotherapists who meet at workshops revolves around what school of therapy one prefers: cognitive behavioral therapy (CBT), acceptance and commitment therapy (ACT), metacognitive therapy (MCT), dialectical behavior therapy (DBT), etc.? The underlying question is really, "What do you believe in?" This procedural pluralism is also reflected when we speak of "waves of therapy" instead of an evolution of psychotherapy. A "third wave" implies that what was previously worked with can be washed away and that after this wave, others will follow, washing over the truths of today (Hayes & Hofmann, 2017).

Toward General Psychotherapy

The process-based approach goes back to the origins of psychotherapy and aims to use process-based functional analysis to make our clients' individual problems understandable and changeable. The goal is *not* to create a new school of therapy but to make schools of therapy and waves of therapy obsolete. A general psychotherapy that focuses on processes and effective factors is not defined by a single dimension, such as "cognitive behavioral," "acceptance and commitment," or "metacognitive," but integrates all biopsychosocial processes that contribute to the development and maintenance of mental health problems. Hayes and Hofmann (2021) advocate eliminating letter combinations and acronyms in the context of psychotherapy as a way to clarify that therapeutic work refers to scientifically based, general psychotherapy. Maybe being able to study "Psychotherapy" similar to studying "Medicine" will contribute to focusing on an overall scientific basis that explores core dimensions of mental suffering and change and prevent psychotherapy from drifting into belief systems. On this scientific foundation it will be possible to focus training on the development of competencies necessary for recognizing and changing these core processes (Rief, 2020).

Process-Based Approaches as a Framework for General Psychotherapy

The process-based approach presented here provides a theoretical and practical framework for a general psychotherapy (Hayes, Hofmann, & Ciarrochi, 2020; Hofmann et al., 2020). It summarizes the theories and findings relevant to general psychotherapy. The main theoretical assumptions are as follows:

- The approach conceptualizes mental disorders as complex networks and thus takes into account the dynamic, nonlinear character of complex systems. By doing this, the approaches overcome the static, not very valid diagnostic categories of the *DSM* and *ICD* (Hayes & Hofmann, 2020; Hofmann et al., 2016).
- The core processes included in the analysis are empirically based vulnerability and response mechanisms.
- The process-based approach follows an ideographic, function-analytical approach. Relevant core processes are assembled into an individual process-based complex network model. This model maps core processes and dynamic interactions between these processes that are responsible for psychopathology (Hofmann et al., 2020).
- Process goals for intervention planning are derived from the complex network model.
- Interventions aim to change the existing network structure. This is achieved either by changing problematic interactions between processes or by promoting adaptive network activity (Hayes et al., 2015).
- Therapeutic interventions are guided by empirically based effect factors (Kazantzis et al., 2018) and interventions that have been shown to be effective in psychotherapy (Klepac et al., 2012).
- A multidimensional model (extended evolutionary metamodel) for diagnosis and therapy serves as a new conceptual basis for analyzing adaptivity/maladaptivity of behavior and change (Hayes, Hofmann, & Wilson, 2020).

Learning to "See" Processes

As mentioned at the beginning of the book, this approach is still in its infancy in terms of practical implementation. Especially if you have been trained as a therapist in the last 20 years, diagnosis-oriented thinking and identifying with individual therapy procedures and methods run deep. We hope that this book can help practitioners to take off the diagnostic and procedural glasses and to look with process-oriented glasses at the individual disorders of clients.

From Metaphor to Calculation

Even if a process-based approach can initially overwhelm, we need to face this complexity in psychotherapy. To do so, we need to develop diagnostic and therapeutic methods to better manage and visualize complexity.

Here it is worth looking at other disciplines that also work with complex models. Meteorologists, financial analysts, biologists, ecologists, and IT specialists have had to further develop their concepts to take into account the complexity they are confronted with. As a result, methods have emerged to visualize and quantify complex processes. This makes it possible to make something complex, such as ecosystem stability, understandable: Climate models explain how individual core processes, such as global warming and CO_2 levels, have an impact on sea level, weather, storm frequency, or restoration costs. Based on such models, interventions can be implemented and monitored worldwide.

In the disciplines mentioned, complex process models are not only used as a metaphor to imagine, for example, a tipping point at which a system tips over and changes irreversibly. With their help, network changes, such as interactions, the change of individual parameters, and even tipping points (e.g., 2-degree limit) can also be calculated mathematically. These model calculations are performed continuously with current and permanently changing data. This makes it possible to continually adjust the forecast of when a self-regulatory state will tip and the current equilibrium will be destabilized.

Thinking into the future of psychotherapy, we need to develop similar methods that will help us map the complexity in psychopathology. These must be able to measure core dimensions so that individual-level interactions can be calculated on this basis and their effects on the person and the environment can be predicted (Hayes et al., 2020). Calculating process dimensions could be used to calculate or foresee when a depressed client tips into a suicidal crisis or when an anorexic client in the process of gaining weight enters a bottleneck in therapy, where the eating-disorder network is highly activated and the risk of dropping out of therapy is high. At the same time the calculated model may give the client and therapist a clue to when the system will stabilize itself and lead to a certain relief.

This has already been achieved to some extent for individual disorders. By continuously calculating intercorrelations, networks can be generated that dynamically describe the development of disorders. The influence of certain process dimensions (e.g., negative affect) on other dimensions of the network is calculated and visualized by the thickness of the arrows. The results are network models as presented in Section 2.8.2 of this book (see Figure 25; Robinaugh et al., 2014). One can see from which nodes many arrows originate, revealing their central role in the formation of the network. However, these models are not static representations but animated network representations where one can observe over time how the nodes and arrow thickness change as they are constantly recalculated. You can literally watch how the network changes. Such computational models can also be used to identify typical patterns that occur before rupture-like changes occur. Thus, a negative feedback loop can intensify from day to day until a critical point is passed at which suicidal thoughts turn into suicidal actions. Steven Hayes is currently working on an application called Mind Graph that calculates the effects of individual processes on reaching a defined therapy goal. In that way, it analyzes on an individual basis which are the relevant core processes for the client in that context that prevent change.

Eliminate Disorder-Specific Approaches?

The adiagnostic approach gives the impression that disorder-specific approaches are superfluous. But this is not true. Disorder-specific therapy research in particular has generated a great deal of process knowledge and contributed to the understanding of disorder mechanisms and treatment approaches (Harvey et al., 2009). Intensive theoretical and practical engagement with a disorder helps to grasp the diverse, underlying core processes in their complexity and individuality and thus gain real expertise. The clinic I (M. S.) work in uses disorder-specific, specialized treatment units, and standardized follow-up assessments show that specialized, disorder-specific treatments demonstrate much higher treatment effects. This can be explained by an increase in the process understanding of a treatment team and the possibility to offer tailored interventions that address core processes of certain disorders (e.g., intense exposure therapy).

First of all, however, we hope that you feel as I did (M. S.) after my sailing course with the 80-year-old sailing instructor. I began to notice previously unnoticed changes in water color, rustling leaves, or wave motion. Over time, seeing these previously hidden phenomena helped me understand the processes behind them. Perhaps you feel the same way about perceiving processes in therapy. Let us know.

References

American Psychiatric Association. (2013). *Diagnostic and statistical manual of mental disorders* (5th ed.). American Psychiatric Publishing.

American Psychological Association. (2016). Revision of Ethical Standard 3.04 of the "Ethical Principles of Psychologists and Code of Conduct" (2002, as amended 2010). *The American Psychologist, 71*(9), 900.

Anestis, M. D., Silva, C., Lavender, J. M., Crosby, R. D., Wonderlich, S. A., Engel, S. E., & Joiner, T. E. (2012). Predicting nonsuicidal self-injury episodes over a discrete period of time in a sample of women diagnosed with bulimia nervosa: An analysis of self-reported trait and ecological momentary assessment based affective lability and previous suicide attempts. *International Journal of Eating Disorders, 45*(6), 808–811.

Antony, M. M., Ledley, D. R., & Heimberg, R. G. (Eds.). (2005). *Improving outcomes and preventing relapse in cognitive-behavioral therapy*. Guilford Press.

Aupperle, R. L., Melrose, A. J., Stein, M. B., & Paulus, M. P. (2012). Executive function and PTSD: Disengaging from trauma. *Neuropharmacology, 62*(2), 686–694. https://doi.org/10.1016/j.neuropharm.2011.02.008

Barlow, D. H. (Ed.). (2014). *Clinical handbook of psychological disorders: A step-by-step treatment manual* (5th ed.). Guilford Press.

Barlow, D. H., Sauer-Zavala, S., Carl, J. R., Bullis, J. R., & Ellard, K. K. (2014). The nature, diagnosis, and treatment of neuroticism: Back to the future. *Clinical Psychological Science, 2*(3), 344–365. https://doi.org/10.1177/2167702613505532

Barthel, A. L., Pinaire, M. A., Curtiss, J. E., Baker, A. W., Brown, M. L., Hoeppner, S. S., Bui, E., Simon, M. N., & Hofmann, S. G. (2020). Anhedonia is central for the association between quality of life, metacognition, sleep, and affective symptoms in generalized anxiety disorder: A complex network analysis. *Journal of Affective Disorders, 277*, 1013–1021. https://doi.org/10.1016/j.jad.2020.08.077

Batra, A., & Bilke-Hentsch, O. (Eds.). (2012). *Praxisbuch Sucht: Therapy of addictive disorders in adolescence and adulthood*. Thieme.

Beck, A. T. (1967). *Depression: Clinical, experimental, and theoretical aspects*. Hoeber Medical Division, Harper & Row.

Bengel, J., & Jerusalem, M. (Eds.). (2009). *Handbook of health and medical psychology*. Hogrefe.

Bennett, R., & Oliver, J. E. (2019). *Acceptance and commitment therapy: 100 key points and techniques*. Routledge. https://doi.org/10.4324/9781351056144

Benoy, C. M. (2019). *Measuring mental flexibility and promoting it in the inclient setting*. Unpublished dissertation, University of Basel.

Berking, M., & Kowalsky, J. (2012). Therapy motivation. In M. Berking & W. Rief (Eds.), *Clinical psychology and psychotherapy for undergraduates* (pp. 13–22). Springer.

Berking, M., & Whitley, B. (2014). *Affect regulation training: A practitioner's manual*. Springer. https://doi.org/10.1007/978-1-4939-1022-9

Bieling, P. J., & Kuyken, W. (2003). Is cognitive case formulation science or science fiction? *Clinical Psychology: Science and Practice, 10*(1), 52–69. https://doi.org/10.1093/clipsy.10.1.52

Bonanno, G. A., & Burton, C. L. (2013). Regulatory flexibility: An individual differences perspective on coping and emotion regulation. *Perspectives on Psychological Science, 8*(6), 591–612. https://doi.org/10.1177/1745691613504116

Bonanno, G. A., Papa, A., Lalande, K., Westphal, M., & Coifman, K. (2004). The importance of being flexible: The ability to both enhance and suppress emotional expression predicts long-term adjustment. *Psychological Science, 15*(7), 482–487. https://doi.org/10.1111/j.0956-7976.2004.00705.x

Bordin, E.S. (1979). The generalizability of the psychoanalytic concept of the working alliance. *Psychotherapy: Theory, Research & Practice, 16*(3), 252. https://doi.org/10.1037/h0085885

Borkovec, T.D., Abel, J.L., & Newman, H. (1995). Effects of psychotherapy on comorbid conditions in generalized anxiety disorder. *Journal of Consulting and Clinical Psychology, 63*(3), 479. https://doi.org/10.1037/0022-006X.63.3.479

Borkovec, T.D., Alcaine, O.M., & Behar, E. (2004). Avoidance theory of worry and generalized anxiety disorder. In R.G. Heimberg, C.L. Turk, & D.S. Mennin (Eds.), *Generalized anxiety disorder: Advances in research and practice* (pp. 77–108). Guilford Press.

Borsboom, D. (2017). A network theory of mental disorders. *World Psychiatry, 16*(1), 5–13. https://doi.org/10.1002/wps.20375

Borsboom, D., & Cramer, A.O. (2013). Network analysis: An integrative approach to the structure of psychopathology. *Annual Review of Clinical Psychology, 9*, 91–121. https://doi.org/10.1146/annurev-clinpsy-050212-185608

Borsboom, D., Cramer, A.O., Schmittmann, V.D., Epskamp, S., & Waldorp, L.J. (2011). The small world of psychopathology. *PloS ONE, 6*(11), e27407. https://doi.org/10.1371/journal.pone.0027407

Bringmann, L.F., Vissers, N., Wichers, M., Geschwind, N., Kuppens, P., Peeters, F., & Tuerlinckx, F. (2013). A network approach to psychopathology: new insights into clinical longitudinal data. *PloS ONE, 8*(4), e60188. https://doi.org/10.1371/journal.pone.0060188

Brown, T.A., & Barlow, D.H. (1992). Comorbidity among anxiety disorders: Implications for treatment and DSM-IV. *Journal of Consulting and Clinical Psychology, 60*(6), 835. https://doi.org/10.1037/0022-006X.60.6.835

Buhr, K., & Dugas, M.J. (2012). Fear of emotions, experiential avoidance, and intolerance of uncertainty in worry and generalized anxiety disorder. *International Journal of Cognitive Therapy, 5*(1), 1–17. https://doi.org/10.1521/ijct.2012.5.1.1

Carver, C.S. (2004). Self-regulation of action and affect. In R.F. Baumeister & K.D. Vohs (Eds.), *Handbook of self-regulation: Research, theory, and applications* (pp. 13–39). Guilford Press.

Cheng, C. (2001). Assessing coping flexibility in real-life and laboratory settings: A multimethod approach. *Journal of Personality and Social Psychology, 80*(5), 814. https://doi.org/10.1037/0022-3514.80.5.814

Cheng, C. (2003). Cognitive and motivational processes underlying coping flexibility: A dual-process model. *Journal of Personality and Social Psychology, 84*(2), 425. https://doi.org/10.1037/0022-3514.84.2.425

Chorpita, B.F., & Barlow, D.H. (1998). The development of anxiety: The role of control in the early environment. *Psychological Bulletin, 124*(1), 3. https://doi.org/10.1037/0033-2909.124.1.3

Cioffi, D., & Holloway, J. (1993). Delayed costs of suppressed pain. *Journal of Personality and Social Psychology, 64*(2), 274. https://doi.org/10.1037/0022-3514.64.2.274

Clark, D.M. (1999). Anxiety disorders: Why they persist and how to treat them. *Behaviour Research and Therapy, 37*(Suppl. 1), S5–S27. https://doi.org/10.1016/S0005-7967(99)00048-0

Clark, D.M., Fairburn, C.G., & Jones, J.V. (1997). The science and practice of cognitive behavior therapy. *Journal of Cognitive Psychotherapy, 11*, 141–144. https://doi.org/10.1891/0889-8391.11.2.141

Clark, D.M., & Wells, A. (1995). A cognitive model of social phobia. In R.G. Heimberg, M.R. Liebowitz, D.A. Hope, & F.R. Schneier (Eds.), *Social phobia: Diagnosis, assessment, and treatment* (pp. 69–93). Guilford Press.

Collimore, K.C., Asmundson, G.J., Taylor, S., & Jang, K.L. (2009). Socially related fears following exposure to trauma: Environmental and genetic influences. *Journal of Anxiety Disorders, 23*(2), 240–246. https://doi.org/10.1016/j.janxdis.2008.07.006

Cramer, A.O., Waldorp, L.J., van der Maas, H.L., & Borsboom, D. (2010). Comorbidity: A network perspective. *Behavioral and Brain Sciences, 33*(2–3), 137. https://doi.org/10.1017/S0140525X09991567

Craske, M.G., & Barlow, D.H. (2014). Panic disorder and agoraphobia. In D.H. Barlow (Ed.), *Clinical handbook of psychological disorders: A step-by-step treatment manual* (pp. 1–61). Guilford Press.

Crowell, S.E., Beauchaine, T.P., McCauley, E., Smith, C.J., Stevens, A.L., & Sylvers, P. (2005). Psychological, autonomic, and serotonergic correlates of parasuicide among adolescent girls. *Development and Psychopathology, 17*(4), 1105–1127. https://doi.org/10.1017/S0954579405050522

Cuijpers, P., van Straten, A., Bohlmeijer, E., Hollon, S. D., & Andersson, G. (2010). The effects of psychotherapy for adult depression are overestimated: A meta-analysis of study quality and effect size. *Psychological Medicine, 40*(2), 211–223. https://doi.org/10.1017/S0033291709006114

Dalgleish, T., Black, M., Johnston, D., & Bevan, A. (2020). Transdiagnostic approaches to mental health problems: Current status and future directions. *Journal of Consulting and Clinical Psychology, 88*(3), 179. https://doi.org/10.1037/ccp0000482

Davidson, R., & Begley, S. (2012). *Why we feel the way we do: How brain structure determines our emotions – and how we can influence them.* Arcana. (Originally published 2012).

De Houwer, J., Barnes-Holmes, D., & Barnes-Holmes, Y. (2018). What is cognition? A functional-cognitive perspective. In S. C. Hayes & S. G. Hofmann (Eds.), *Process-based CBT: The science and core clinical competencies of cognitive behavioral therapy* (pp. 119–136). New Harbinger.

Deacon, B. J. (2013). The biomedical model of mental disorder: A critical analysis of its validity, utility, and effects on psychotherapy research. *Clinical Psychology Review, 33*(7), 846–861. https://doi.org/10.1016/j.cpr.2012.09.007

Deci, E. L., & Ryan, R. M. (2008). Self-determination theory: A macrotheory of human motivation, development, and health. *Canadian Psychology/Psychologie Canadienne, 49*(3), 182. https://doi.org/10.1037/a0012801

Dixon, M. R., & Rehfeldt, R. A. (2018). Core behavioral processes. In S. C. Hayes & S. G. Hofmann (Eds.), *Process-based CBT: The science and core clinical competencies of cognitive behavioral therapy* (pp. 101–117). New Harbinger.

Dougher, M. J., Hamilton, D. A., Fink, B. C., & Harrington, J. (2007). Transformation of the discriminative and eliciting functions of generalized relational stimuli. *Journal of the Experimental Analysis of Behavior, 88*(2), 179–197. https://doi.org/10.1901/jeab.2007.45-05

Dugas, M. J., Buhr, K., & Ladouceur, R. (2004). The role of intolerance of uncertainty in etiology and maintenance. In R. G. Heimberg, C. L. Turk, & D. S. Mennin (Eds.), *Generalized anxiety disorder: Advances in research and practice* (pp. 143–163). Guilford Press.

Egan, S. J., Wade, T. D., & Shafran, R. (2011). Perfectionism as a transdiagnostic process: A clinical review. *Clinical Psychology Review, 31*(2), 203–212. https://doi.org/10.1016/j.cpr.2010.04.009

Ekman, P., & Friesen, W. V. (1982). Felt, false, and miserable smiles. *Journal of Nonverbal Behavior, 6*(4), 238–252. https://doi.org/10.1007/BF00987191

Ellis, A. (1989). Rational psychotherapy. *TACD Journal, 17*(1), 67–80. https://doi.org/10.1080/1046171X.1989.12034348

Eysenck, M. W., Derakshan, N., Santos, R., & Calvo, M. G. (2007). Anxiety and cognitive performance: Attentional control theory. *Emotion, 7*(2), 336. https://doi.org/10.1037/1528-3542.7.2.336

Fisher, A. J., Medaglia, J. D., & Jeronimus, B. F. (2018). Lack of group-to-individual generalizability is a threat to human subjects research. *Proceedings of the National Academy of Sciences, 115*(27), E6106–E6115. https://doi.org/10.1073/pnas.1711978115

Frank, R. I., & Davidson, J. (2014). *The transdiagnostic road map to case formulation and treatment planning: Practical guidance for clinical decision making.* New Harbinger.

Fried, E. I. (2015). Problematic assumptions have slowed down depression research: Why symptoms, not syndromes are the way forward. *Frontiers in Psychology, 6*, 309. https://doi.org/10.3389/fpsyg.2015.00309

Fried, E. I., & Nesse, R. M. (2015). Depression sum-scores don't add up: Why analyzing specific depression symptoms is essential. *BMC Medicine, 13*(1), 1–11. https://doi.org/10.1186/s12916-015-0325-4

Frost, R. O., Marten, P., Lahart, C., & Rosenblate, R. (1990). The dimensions of perfectionism. *Cognitive Therapy and Research, 14*, 449–468. https://doi.org/10.1007/BF01172967

Gehrman, P. R., Pfeiffenberger, C., & Byrne, E. M. (2013). The role of genes in the insomnia phenotype. *Sleep Medicine Clinics, 8*(3), 323–331. https://doi.org/10.1016/j.jsmc.2013.04.005

Gilbert, P. (Ed.). (2005). *Compassion: Conceptualisations, research and use in psychotherapy.* Routledge.

Gloster, A. T., & Karekla, M. (2020). A multilevel, multimethod approach to testing and refining intervention targets. In S. C. Hayes & S. G. Hofmann (Eds.), *Beyond the DSM: Toward a process-based alternative for diagnosis and mental health treatment* (pp. 225–251). Context Press.

Gohm, C. L., & Clore, G. L. (2000). Individual differences in emotional experience: Mapping available scales to processes. *Personality and Social Psychology Bulletin, 26*(6), 679–697. https://doi.org/10.1177/0146167200268004

Grawe, K. (1995). Outline of a general psychotherapy. *Psychotherapist, 40*(3), 130–145.

Grawe, K. (1998). *Psychological therapy*. Hogrefe.

Grawe, K., Donati, R., & Bernauer, F. (1994). *Psychotherapy in transition: From denomination to profession.* Göttingen: Hogrefe.

Gross, R. (2015). *Psychology: The science of mind and behavior* (7th ed.). Hodder Education.

Grossmann, K., & Grossmann, K. (2004). *Attachments: The fabric of psychological security*. Klett-Cotta.

Guy, W., & Ban, T. A. (1982). *The AMDP system: Manual for the assessment and documentation of psychopathology*. Springer. https://doi.org/10.1007/978-3-642-68405-0

Guze, S. B. (1992). *Why psychiatry is a branch of medicine.* Oxford University Press.

Harvey, A. G., Watkins, E., Mansell, W., & Shafran, R. (2009). *Cognitive behavioural processes across psychological disorders: A transdiagnostic approach to research and treatment*. Oxford University Press.

Hayes, A. M. (2015). Facilitating emotional processing in depression: The application of exposure principles. *Current Opinion in Psychology, 4*, 61–66. https://doi.org/10.1016/j.copsyc.2015.03.032

Hayes, A. M., & Andrews, L. A. (2020). What a complex systems perspective can contribute to process-based assessment and psychotherapy. In S. C. Hayes & S. G. Hofmann (Eds.), *Beyond the DSM: Toward a process-based alternative for diagnosis and mental health treatment* (pp. 165–198). Context Press.

Hayes, A. M., Yasinski, C., Barnes, J. B., & Bockting, C. L. (2015). Network destabilization and transition in depression: New methods for studying the dynamics of therapeutic change. *Clinical Psychology Review, 41*, 27–39. https://doi.org/10.1016/j.cpr.2015.06.007

Hayes, S. C. (2004). Acceptance and commitment therapy, relational frame theory, and the third wave of behavioral and cognitive therapies. *Behavior Therapy, 35*(4), 639–665. https://doi.org/10.1016/S0005-7894(04)80013-3

Hayes, S. C., Barnes-Holmes, D., & Roche, B. (2001). *Relational frame theory: A post-Skinnerian account of human language and cognition*. Springer. https://doi.org/10.1007/b108413

Hayes, S. C., & Hofmann, S. G. (2017). The third wave of CBT and the rise of process-based care. *World Psychiatry, 16*, 245–246. https://doi.org/10.1002/wps.20442

Hayes, S. C., & Hofmann, S. G. (2018a). Future directions in CBT and evidence-based therapy. In S. C. Hayes & S. G. Hofmann (Eds.), *Process-based CBT: The science and core clinical competencies of cognitive behavioral therapy* (pp. 427–435). New Harbinger.

Hayes, S. C., & Hofmann, S. G. (Eds.). (2018b). *Process-based CBT: The science and core clinical competencies of cognitive behavioral therapy*. New Harbinger.

Hayes, S. C., & Hofmann, S. G. (Eds.). (2020). *Beyond the DSM: Toward a process-based alternative for diagnosis and mental health treatment*. Context Press.

Hayes, S. C., & Hofmann, S. G. (2021). "Third-wave" cognitive and behavioral therapies and the emergence of a process-based approach to intervention in psychiatry. *World Psychiatry, 20*, 363–375. https://doi.org/10.1002/wps.20884

Hayes, S. C., Hofmann, S. G., & Ciarrochi, J. (2020). A process-based approach to psychological diagnosis and treatment: The conceptual and treatment utility of an extended evolutionary meta model. *Clinical Psychology Review, 82*, 101908. https://doi.org/10.1016/j.cpr.2020.101908

Hayes, S. C., Hofmann, S. G., & Ciarrochi, J. (2023). The idionomic future of cognitive behavioral therapy: What stands out from criticisms of ACT development. *Behavior Therapy, 54*(6), 1036–1063. https://doi.org/10.1016/j.beth.2023.07.011

Hayes, S. C., Hofmann, S. G., & Wilson, D. S. (2020). Clinical psychology is an applied evolutionary science. *Clinical Psychology Review, 81*, 101892. https://doi.org/10.1016/j.cpr.2020.101892

Hayes, S. C., Monestès, J. L., & Wilson, D. S. (2018). Evolutionary principles for applied psychology. In S. C. Hayes & S. G. Hofmann (Eds.), *Process-based CBT: The science and core clinical competencies of cognitive behavioral therapy* (pp. 155–171). New Harbinger.

Hayes, S. C., Strosahl, K. D., & Wilson, K. G. (2009). *Acceptance and commitment therapy*. American Psychological Association.

Hayes, S. C., Wilson, K. G., Gifford, E. V., Follette, V. M., & Strosahl, K. (1996). Experiential avoidance and behavioral disorders: A functional dimensional approach to diagnosis and treatment. *Journal of Consulting and Clinical Psychology, 64*(6), 1152. https://doi.org/10.1037/0022-006X.64.6.1152

Heidenreich, T., & Michalak, J. (Eds.). (2013). *The "third wave" of behavior therapy. Foundations and practice*. Beltz.

Henning-Fast, K., & Markowitsch, H. J. (2010). Neuropsychology of posttraumatic stress disorder (PTSD). In S. Lautenbacher & S. Gauggel (Eds.), *Neuropsychology of mental disorders* (2nd ed., fully updated, pp. 241–284). Springer.

Herpertz, S. C., Dietrich, T. M., Wenning, B., Krings, T., Erberich, S. G., Willmes, K., Thron, A. & Sass, H. (2001). Evidence of abnormal amygdala functioning in borderline personality disorder: a functional MRI study. *Biological Psychiatry, 50*(4), 292–298. https://doi.org/10.1016/S0006-3223(01)01075-7

Hofmann, S. G. (2019). *Emotion in therapy. From science to practice*. Guilford.

Hofmann, S. G., Curtiss, J. E., & Hayes, S. C. (2020). Beyond linear mediation: Toward a dynamic network approach to study treatment processes. *Clinical Psychology Review, 76*, 101824. https://doi.org/10.1016/j.cpr.2020.101824

Hofmann, S. G., Curtiss, J., & McNally, R. J. (2016). A complex network perspective on clinical science. *Perspectives on Psychological Science, 11*(5), 597–605. https://doi.org/10.1177/1745691616639283

Hofmann, S. G., & Hayes, S. C. (2018). The history and current status of CBT as an evidence-based therapy. In S. C. Hayes & S. G. Hofmann (Eds.), *Process-based CBT: The science and core clinical competencies of cognitive behavioral therapy* (pp. 7–22). New Harbinger.

Hofmann, S. G., & Hayes, S. C. (2019). The future of intervention science: Process-based therapy. *Clinical Psychological Science, 7*, 37–50. https://doi.org/10.1177/2167702618772296

Hofmann, S. G., Heering, S., Sawyer, A. T., & Asnaani, A. (2009). How to handle anxiety: The effects of reappraisal, acceptance, and suppression strategies on anxious arousal. *Behaviour Research and Therapy, 47*(5), 389–394. https://doi.org/10.1016/j.brat.2009.02.010

Horvath, A. O., & Bedi, R. P. (2002). The alliance. In J. C. Norcross (Ed.), *Psychotherapy relationships that work: Therapists contributions and responsiveness to clients* (pp. 37–69). Oxford University Press.

Hoyer, J., & Gloster, A. T. (2013). Measuring psychological flexibility: The acceptance and action questionnaire II (FAH-II). *Behavior Therapy, 23*(1), 42–44.

Insel, T., Cuthbert, B., Garvey, M., Heinssen, R., Pine, D. S., Quinn, K., Sanislow, C., & Wang, P. (2010). Research domain criteria (RDoC): Toward a new classification framework for research on mental disorders. *American Journal of Psychiatry, 167*(7), 748–751. https://doi.org/10.1176/appi.ajp.2010.09091379

James, W. (1983). *Essays in psychology* (Vol. 13). Harvard University Press. (Originally published 1890).

Jose, A., & Goldfried, M. (2008). A transtheoretical approach to case formulation. *Cognitive and Behavioral Practice, 15*(2), 212–222. https://doi.org/10.1016/j.cbpra.2007.02.009

Kanfer, F. H., Reinecker, H., & Schmelzer, D. (2006). *Self-management therapy*. Springer.

Kazantzis, N., Luong, H. K., Usatoff, A. S., Impala, T., Yew, R. Y., & Hofmann, S. G. (2018). The processes of cognitive behavioral therapy: A review of meta-analyses. *Cognitive Therapy and Research, 42*(4), 349–357. https://doi.org/10.1007/s10608-018-9920-y

Kendall, P. C., Howard, B. L., & Hays, R. C. (1989). Self-referent speech and psychopathology: The balance of positive and negative thinking. *Cognitive Therapy and Research, 13*(6), 583–598. https://doi.org/10.1007/BF01176069

Keough, M. E., Riccardi, C. J., Timpano, K. R., Mitchell, M. A., & Schmidt, N. B. (2010). Anxiety symptomatology: The association with distress tolerance and anxiety sensitivity. *Behavior Therapy, 41*(4), 567–574. https://doi.org/10.1016/j.beth.2010.04.002

Kessler, R. C., McGonagle, K. A., Zhao, S., Nelson, C. B., Hughes, M., Eshleman, S., Wittchen, H. U., & Kendler, K. S. (1994). Lifetime and 12-month prevalence of DSM-III-R psychiatric disorders in the United States: Results from the National Comorbidity Survey. *Archives of General Psychiatry, 51*(1), 8–19. https://doi.org/10.1001/archpsyc.1994.03950010008002

Kircanski, K., Lieberman, M.D., & Craske, M.G. (2012). Feelings into words: Contributions of language to exposure therapy. *Psychological Science, 23*(10), 1086–1091. https://doi.org/10.1177/09567976 12443830

Klepac, R.K., Ronan, G.F., Andrasik, F., Arnold, K.D., Belar, C.D., Berry, S.L., Christoff, K.A., Craighead, L.W., Dougher, M.J., Dowd, E.T., Herbert, J.D., McFarr, L.M., Rizvi, S.L., Sauer, E.M., & Strauman, T.J. (2012). Guidelines for cognitive behavioral training within doctoral psychology programs in the United States: Report of the Inter-organizational Task Force on Cognitive and Behavioral Psychology Doctoral Education. *Behavior Therapy, 43*(4), 687–697.

Lambert, M.J. (2010). *Prevention of treatment failure: The use of measuring, monitoring, and feedback in clinical practice.* American Psychological Association. https://doi.org/10.1037/12141-000

Lazarus, R.S. (1974). Psychological stress and coping in adaptation and illness. *The International Journal of Psychiatry in Medicine, 5*(4), 321–333. https://doi.org/10.2190/T43T-84P3-QDUR-7RTP

Linehan, M.M. (1993). Dialectical behavior therapy for treatment of borderline personality disorder: Implications for the treatment of substance abuse. *NIDA Research Monograph, 137*, 201–216.

Linehan, M.M., Bohus, M., & Lynch, T.R. (2007). Dialectical behavior therapy for pervasive emotion dysregulation. In J.J. Gross (Ed.), *Handbook of emotion regulation* (pp. 581–605). Guilford Press.

Macneil, C.A., Hasty, M.K., Conus, P., & Berk, M. (2012). Is diagnosis enough to guide interventions in mental health? Using case formulation in clinical practice. *BMC Medicine, 10*(1), 111. https://doi.org/10.1186/1741-7015-10-111

Malta, L.S., Wyka, K.E., Giosan, C., Jayasinghe, N., & Difede, J. (2009). Numbing symptoms as predictors of unremitting posttraumatic stress disorder. *Journal of Anxiety Disorders, 23*(2), 223–229. https://doi.org/10.1016/j.janxdis.2008.07.004

Margraf, M., & Berking, M. (2005). With a "why" in your heart, almost any "how" can be endured: Psychotherapeutic resolution support. *Behavior Therapy, 15*(4), 254–261.

Marroquín, B. (2011). Interpersonal emotion regulation as a mechanism of social support in depression. *Clinical Psychology Review, 31*(8), 1276–1290. https://doi.org/10.1016/j.cpr.2011.09.005

Mayer, J.D., & Salovey, P. (1997). What is emotional intelligence? In P. Salovey & D.J. Sluyter (Eds.), *Emotional development and emotional intelligence: Educational implications* (pp. 3–31). Basic Books.

McCullough, J.P., Jr. (2003). Treatment for chronic depression: Cognitive behavioral analysis system of psychotherapy (CBASP). *Journal of Psychotherapy Integration, 13*(3–4), 241–263. https://doi.org/10.1037/1053-0479.13.3-4.241

McEwen, B.S. (2003). Mood disorders and allostatic load. *Biological Psychiatry, 54*(3), 200–207. https://doi.org/10.1016/S0006-3223(03)00177-X

McHugh, R.K., Murray, H.W., & Barlow, D.H. (2009). Balancing fidelity and adaptation in the dissemination of empirically-supported treatments: The promise of transdiagnostic interventions. *Behaviour Research and Therapy, 47*(11), 946–953. https://doi.org/10.1016/j.brat.2009.07.005

McHugh, R.K., Reynolds, E.K., Leyro, T.M., & Otto, M.W. (2013). An examination of the association of distress intolerance and emotion regulation with avoidance. *Cognitive Therapy and Research, 37*(2), 363–367. https://doi.org/10.1007/s10608-012-9463-6

McKey, Z. (2019). *Think in systems: The theory and practice of strategic planning, problem solving, and creating lasting results – Complexity made simple.* CreateSpace Independent Publishing Platform.

McNally, R.J. (2016). Can network analysis transform psychopathology? *Behavior Research and Therapy, 86*, 95–104. https://doi.org/10.1016/j.brat.2016.06.006

McNally, R.J., Robinaugh, D.J., Wu, G.W., Wang, L., Deserno, M.K., & Borsboom, D. (2015). Mental disorders as causal systems: A network approach to posttraumatic stress disorder. *Clinical Psychological Science, 3*(6), 836–849. https://doi.org/10.1177/2167702614553230

Meadows, D.H. (2008). *Thinking in systems: A primer.* Chelsea Green Publishing.

Miklowitz, D.J., & Johnson, S.L. (2006). The psychopathology and treatment of bipolar disorder. *Annual Review of Clinical Psychology, 2*, 199–235. https://doi.org/10.1146/annurev.clinpsy.2.022305.095332

Molenaar, P.C. (2004). A manifesto on psychology as idiographic science: Bringing the person back into scientific psychology, this time forever. *Measurement, 2*(4), 201–218.

Montada, L. (1995). Mental development from Jean Piaget's perspective. In R. Rolf & L. Montada, *Developmental psychology* (2nd, revised ed., pp. 518–560). Beltz.

Mor, N., & Winquist, J. (2002). Self-focused attention and negative affect: A meta-analysis. *Psychological Bulletin, 128*(4), 638. https://doi.org/10.1037/0033-2909.128.4.638

Myers, D. G. (2000). Feeling good about Fredrickson's positive emotions. *Prevention & Treatment, 3*(1), Article 2c. https://doi.org/10.1037/1522-3736.3.1.32c

Neisser, U. (1994). Multiple systems: A new approach to cognitive theory. *European Journal of Cognitive Psychology, 6*(3), 225–241. https://doi.org/10.1080/09541449408520146

Nelson, B., McGorry, P. D., Wichers, M., Wigman, J. T., & Hartmann, J. A. (2017). Moving from static to dynamic models of the onset of mental disorder: A review. *JAMA Psychiatry, 74*(5), 528–534. https://doi.org/10.1001/jamapsychiatry.2017.0001

Nezu, A. M., Nezu, C. M., & Lombardo, E. R. (2004). *Cognitive-behavioral case formulation and treatment design: A problem-solving approach.* Springer Publishing Company.

Nye, A., Delgadillo, J., & Barkham, M. (2023). Efficacy of personalized psychological interventions: A systematic review and meta-analysis. *Journal of Consulting and Clinical Psychology, 91*(7), 389–397. https://doi.org/10.1037/ccp0000820

Papa, A., Emerson, M., & Epstein, E. (2018). Emotions and emotion regulation. In S. C. Hayes & S. G. Hofmann (Eds.), *Process-based CBT: The science and core clinical competencies of cognitive behavioral therapy* (pp. 137–151). New Harbinger.

Persons, J. B. (1989). *Cognitive therapy in practice: A case formulation approach.* Norton.

Petermann, F., & Ulrich, F. (2019). Developmental psychopathology. In S. Schneider & J. Margraf (Eds.), *Textbook of behavior therapy* (Vol. 3, pp. 23–40). Springer.

Porges, S. W., & Lewis, G. F. (2010). The polyvagal hypothesis: Common mechanisms mediating autonomic regulation, vocalizations and listening. In S. Brudzynski (Ed.), *Handbook of mammalian vocalization: An integrative neuroscience approach* (pp. 255–264). Academic Press. https://doi.org/10.1016/B978-0-12-374593-4.00025-5

Potreck-Rose, F. (2006). Psychotherapeutic interventions to strengthen self-esteem. *PiD – Psychotherapie im Dialog, 7*(3), 313–317. https://doi.org/10.1055/s-2006-940070

Prochaska, J. O., & DiClemente, C. C. (1983). Stages and processes of self-change of smoking: Toward an integrative model of change. *Journal of Consulting and Clinical Psychology, 51*(3), 390–395. https://doi.org/10.1037/0022-006X.51.3.390

Pyszczynski, T., & Greenberg, J. (1987). Self-regulatory perseveration and the depressive self-focusing style: A self-awareness theory of reactive depression. *Psychological Bulletin, 102*(1), 122–138. https://doi.org/10.1037/0033-2909.102.1.122

Richards, J. M., Stipelman, B. A., Bornovalova, M. A., Daughters, S. B., Sinha, R., & Lejuez, C. W. (2011). Biological mechanisms underlying the relationship between stress and smoking: State of the science and directions for future work. *Biological Psychology, 88*(1), 1–12. https://doi.org/10.1016/j.biopsycho.2011.06.009

Reiss, S. (1991). Expectancy model of fear, anxiety, and panic. *Clinical Psychology Review, 11*(2), 141–153. https://doi.org/10.1016/0272-7358(91)90092-9

Rief, W (2020). Expectations and related cognitive domains: Implications for classification and therapy. In S. C. Hayes & S. G. Hofmann (Eds.), *Beyond the DSM: Toward a process-based alternative for diagnosis and mental health treatment* (pp. 97–115). Context Press.

Robinaugh, D. J., LeBlanc, N. J., Vuletich, H. A., & McNally, R. J. (2014). Network analysis of persistent complex bereavement disorder in conjugally bereaved adults. *Journal of Abnormal Psychology, 123*(3), 510–522. https://doi.org/10.1037/abn0000002

Robinaugh, D. J., Millner, A. J., & McNally, R. J. (2016). Identifying highly influential nodes in the complicated grief network. *Journal of Abnormal Psychology, 125*(6), 747–757. https://doi.org/10.1037/abn0000181

Rozanski, A., & Kubzansky, L. D. (2005). Psychologic functioning and physical health: A paradigm of flexibility. *Psychosomatic Medicine, 67*, S47–S53. https://doi.org/10.1097/01.psy.0000164253.69550.49

Salkovskis, P., Shafran, R., Rachman, S., & Freeston, M.H. (1999). Multiple pathways to inflated responsibility beliefs in obsessional problems: Possible origins and implications for therapy and research. *Behavior Research and Therapy, 37*(11), 1055–1072. https://doi.org/10.1016/S0005-7967(99)00063-7

Scheffer, M., Carpenter, S.R., Lenton, T.M., Bascompte, J., Brock, W., Dakos, V., van de Koppel, I.A., Levin, S.A., van Nes, E.H., Pascual, M., & Vandermeer, J. (2012). Anticipating critical transitions. *Science, 338*(6105), 344–348.

Scherer, K.R. (2009). The dynamic architecture of emotion: Evidence for the component process model. *Cognition and Emotion, 23*(7), 1307–1351. https://doi.org/10.1080/02699930902928969

Scherer, K.R., Schorr, A., & Johnstone, T. (Eds.). (2001). *Appraisal processes in emotion: Theory, methods, research*. Oxford University Press.

Schwartz, R.M. (1997). Consider the simple screw: Cognitive science, quality improvement, and psychotherapy. *Journal of Consulting and Clinical Psychology, 65*(6), 970–983. https://doi.org/10.1037/0022-006X.65.6.970

Sheppes, G., & Gross, J.J. (2012). Emotion regulation effectiveness: What works when. In H. Tennen, J. Suls, & I.B. Weiner (Eds.), *Handbook of psychology, Volume 5: Personality and social psychology* (2nd ed., pp. 391–405). Wiley.

Sheppes, G., Suri, G., & Gross, J.J. (2015). Emotion regulation and psychopathology. *Annual Review of Clinical Psychology, 11*, 379–405. https://doi.org/10.1146/annurev-clinpsy-032814-112739

Slavich, G.M., & Cole, S.W. (2013). The emerging field of human social genomics. *Clinical Psychological Science, 1*(3), 331–348. https://doi.org/10.1177/2167702613478594

Soares, I., Dias, P., Klein, J., & Machado, P.P. (2008). Attachment and eating disorders. In B. Strauss (Ed.), *Attachment and psychopathology* (pp. 188–211). Klett-Cotta.

Solanto, M.V. (2011). *Cognitive-behavioral therapy for adult ADHD: Targeting executive dysfunction*. Guilford Press.

Spijker, J., van Straten, A., Bockting, C.L., Meeuwissen, J.A., & van Balkom, A.J. (2013). Psychotherapy, antidepressants, and their combination for chronic major depressive disorder: A systematic review. *The Canadian Journal of Psychiatry, 58*(7), 386–392. https://doi.org/10.1177/070674371305800703

Stangier, U. (2019). Process-based cognitive behavioral therapy: Integrating cognitive behavioral therapy and third wave from the perspective of process orientation. *Psychotherapeutenjournal, 18*(3), 236–244.

Steil, R., & Ehlers, A. (2000). Dysfunctional meaning of posttraumatic intrusions in chronic PTSD. *Behaviour Research and Therapy, 38*(6), 537–558. https://doi.org/10.1016/S0005-7967(99)00069-8

Sterling, P. (2004). Principles of allostasis: Optimal design, predictive regulation, pathophysiology, and rational therapeutics. In J. Schulkin (Ed.), *Allostasis, homeostasis, and the costs of physiological adaptation* (pp. 17–64). Cambridge University Press. https://doi.org/10.1017/CBO9781316257081.004

Strauss, B. (Ed.). (2008). *Attachment and psychopathology*. Klett-Cotta.

Stuewig, J., Tangney, J.P., Heigel, C., Harty, L., & McCloskey, L. (2010). Shaming, blaming, and maiming: Functional links among the moral emotions, externalization of blame, and aggression. *Journal of Research in Personality, 44*(1), 91–102. https://doi.org/10.1016/j.jrp.2009.12.005

Suárez, L.M., Bennett, S.M., Goldstein, C.R., & Barlow, D.H. (2009). Understanding anxiety disorders from a "triple vulnerability" framework. In M.M. Antony & M.B. Stein (Eds.), *Oxford handbook of anxiety and related disorders* (pp. 153–172). Oxford University Press.

Suvak, M.K., Litz, B.T., Sloan, D.M., Zanarini, M.C., Barrett, L.F., & Hofmann, S.G. (2011). Emotional granularity and borderline personality disorder. *Journal of Abnormal Psychology, 120*(2), 414–426. https://doi.org/10.1037/a0021808

Szasz, P.L., Szentagotai, A., & Hofmann, S.G. (2011). The effect of emotion regulation strategies on anger. *Behaviour Research and Therapy, 49*(2), 114–119. https://doi.org/10.1016/j.brat.2010.11.011

Szasz, P.L., Szentagotai, A., & Hofmann, S.G. (2012). Effects of emotion regulation strategies on smoking craving, attentional bias, and task persistence. *Behaviour Research and Therapy, 50*(5), 333–340. https://doi.org/10.1016/j.brat.2012.02.010

Taylor, G. J., & Bagby, R. M. (2000). An overview of the alexithymia construct. In R. Bar-On & J. D. A. Parker (Eds.), *The handbook of emotional intelligence: Theory, development, assessment, and application at home, school, and in the workplace* (p. 40–67). Jossey-Bass.

Tee, J., & Kazantzis, N. (2011). Collaborative empiricism in cognitive therapy: A definition and theory for the relationship construct. *Clinical Psychology: Science and Practice, 18*(1), 47–61. https://doi.org/10.1111/j.1468-2850.2010.01234.x

Thiel, A., Jacobi, C., Horstmann, S., Paul, T., Nutzinger, D. O., & Schüßler, G. (1997). A German language version of the Eating Disorder Inventory EDI-2. *PPmP: Psychotherapy Psychosomatics Medical Psychology, 47*(9–10), 365–376.

Thomas, A., & Chess, S. (1980). *Temperament and development: On the emergence of the individual.* Ferdinand Enke.

Tugade, M. M., Fredrickson, B. L., & Feldman Barrett, L. (2004). Psychological resilience and positive emotional granularity: Examining the benefits of positive emotions on coping and health. *Journal of Personality, 72*(6), 1161–1190. https://doi.org/10.1111/j.1467-6494.2004.00294.x

Turk, C. L., Heimberg, R. G., Luterek, J. A., Mennin, D. S., & Fresco, D. M. (2005). Emotion dysregulation in generalized anxiety disorder: A comparison with social anxiety disorder. *Cognitive Therapy and Research, 29*(1), 89–106. https://doi.org/10.1007/s10608-005-1651-1

Utschig, A. C., Presnell, K., Madeley, M. C., & Smits, J. A. (2010). An investigation of the relationship between fear of negative evaluation and bulimic psychopathology. *Eating Behaviors, 11*(4), 231–238. https://doi.org/10.1016/j.eatbeh.2010.05.003

Vaidyanathan, U., Pratap, A., Lattie, E. G., & Galatzerlevy, I. (2020). Aligning real-world evidence collection with the NIMH research domain criteria (RDoC) for assessing mental health disorders [Abstract]. *Annals of Behavioral Medicine, 54*(Suppl. 1), 183.

Watson, D. (2004). Stability versus change, dependability versus error: Issues in the assessment of personality over time. *Journal of Research in Personality, 38*(4), 319–350. https://doi.org/10.1016/j.jrp.2004.03.001

Webb, T. L., Miles, E., & Sheeran, P. (2012). Dealing with feeling: A meta-analysis of the effectiveness of strategies derived from the process model of emotion regulation. *Psychological Bulletin, 138*(4), 775–808. https://doi.org/10.1037/a0027600

Wegner, D. M., Schneider, D. J., Carter, S. R., & White, T. L. (1987). Paradoxical effects of thought suppression. *Journal of Personality and Social Psychology, 53*(1), 5–13. https://doi.org/10.1037/0022-3514.53.1.5

Weiss, D. S., & Marmar, C. (1997). The impact of events scale-revised. In J. P. Wilson & T. M. Keane (Eds.), *Assessing psychological trauma and PTDS* (pp. 399–411). Guilford Press.

Wells, A. (2009). *Metacognitive therapy for anxiety and depression.* Guilford Press.

Wells, A., & Davies, M. (1994). The thought control questionnaire: A measure of individual differences in the control of unwanted thoughts. *Behaviour Research and Therapy, 32,* 871–878. https://doi.org/10.1016/0005-7967(94)90168-6

Wood, W. (2019). *Good habits, bad habits: The science of making positive changes that stick.* Pan.

Appendix

Worksheets 1–18

Worksheet 1:   Guide to a Process-Based Anamnesis

Worksheet 2:   Hypothesis Sheet on Relevant Core Processes

Worksheet 3:   Checklist: Vulnerability Mechanisms

Worksheet 4:   Checklist: Problematic Response Mechanisms

Worksheet 5:   Process-Based Functional Analysis: Support Questions

Worksheet 6:   Process-Based Functional Analysis: Support Questions

Worksheet 7:   Questions for Relatives About the Development of the Disease

Worksheet 8:   Process-Based Assessment of Psychopathology

Worksheet 9:   Emotional Stress Test: 3-Hour Monitor (5-Minute Intervals)

Worksheet 10: Emotion-Monitor Over the Course of a Day

Worksheet 11:   Monitoring Emotions on a Daily Basis

Worksheet 12: 24/7 Monitor

Worksheet 13: Process-Based Diathesis Model

Worksheet 14: Evaluating Adaptivity Through the Extended Evolutionary Metamodel (Hayes & Hofmann, 2020)

Worksheet 15: Motivation: Building up Motivation to Actively Change

Worksheet 16: Cost-Benefit Analysis for Treatment

Worksheet 17: Evidence-Based Treatment Strategies (Kazantzis et al., 2018)

Worksheet 18: Standard Psychotherapeutic Procedures for Targeted Interventions

Appendix 187

Worksheet 1 (page 1/7)

Guide to a Process-Based Anamnesis

1. Spontaneously reported symptomatology
What brings you to therapy?
What are you suffering from?

2. External triggering events
Which external events/stressors/problems have triggered your problems?
Which ones weigh particularly heavily on you?

© 2024 Schoen Clinic Bad Staffelstein, Germany. Reprinted with permission.

This page may be reproduced by the purchaser for personal/clinical use.
From: Michael Svitak and Stefan G. Hofmann: *A Process-Based Approach to CBT* (ISBN 978-0-88937-628-1)
© 2024 Hogrefe Publishing

See p. 213 for instructions on how to obtain the full-sized worksheets as printable PDFs.

188   Appendix

Worksheet 1 (page 2/7)

Guide to a Process-Based Anamnesis

3. Internal coping demands

What is it exactly that you are struggling with? What makes it so threatening/unbearable for you?
Which feelings are difficult to bear? Which thoughts are difficult to endure?
What difficulties does it create in your relationship with others?
What physical effects does it cause you? Or which do you fear?

_____

_____

_____

_____

_____

_____

_____

_____

_____

4. Vulnerability mechanisms

You have overcome many other difficulties in life. What makes this situation so difficult for you?
What sore point does the situation hit?
What are other people good at that makes them cope better with this situation?
Individual vulnerability mechanisms can be explicitly queried and discussed with the help of the Checklist: Vulnerability Mechanisms (Worksheet 3)

_____

_____

_____

_____

_____

_____

_____

_____

_____

This page may be reproduced by the purchaser for personal/clinical use.
From: Michael Svitak and Stefan G. Hofmann: *A Process-Based Approach to CBT* (ISBN 978-0-88937-628-1)
© 2024 Hogrefe Publishing

See p. 213 for instructions on how to obtain the full-sized worksheets as printable PDFs.

Appendix 189

Worksheet 1 (page 3/7)

Guide to a Process-Based Anamnesis

5. Response mechanisms
You had to react to a demanding situation: cognitively, emotionally and through actions. Let's take a closer look.

5.1 Cognitive response

Content: what the person thought
What did you think? What else?
What conclusions did you draw?
What do these thoughts mean to you?

_____

_____

_____

_____

_____

_____

_____

Process of thinking triggered by the events
How did you continue to respond to the situation mentally?
Did your thinking change (fusion, rumination, circling of thoughts, dissociation)?
How would you describe your thinking? How long were you in this thinking mode?
Did the thinking help? Benefits/costs?
How absorbed were you in your thoughts (0–100%)?
Were the thoughts purposeful or were they spinning in circles?
Did you try not to think or change the thoughts? What happened?

_____

_____

_____

_____

_____

_____

_____

_____

This page may be reproduced by the purchaser for personal/clinical use.
From: Michael Svitak and Stefan G. Hofmann: *A Process-Based Approach to CBT* (ISBN 978-0-88937-628-1)
© 2024 Hogrefe Publishing

See p. 213 for instructions on how to obtain the full-sized worksheets as printable PDFs.

190   **Appendix**

Worksheet 1 (page 4/7)

Guide to a Process-Based Anamnesis

5.2 Emotional response

Content: what the person felt
What feelings did the situation trigger in you?
Did these feelings trigger any other feelings?
Which ones are particularly unpleasant for you?

_____

_____

_____

_____

_____

_____

_____

_____

_____

Processes dealing with the regulation of emotions
How did you react to these feelings? How did you deal with them?
Did you do anything to lessen the feelings? Did it help? Or did it make no difference or make the feelings worse?
And when the feelings kept coming, what did you do?
Query individual strategies: alcohol, drugs, exercise, eating.

_____

_____

_____

_____

_____

_____

_____

_____

_____

_____

This page may be reproduced by the purchaser for personal/clinical use.
From: Michael Svitak and Stefan G. Hofmann: *A Process-Based Approach to CBT* (ISBN 978-0-88937-628-1)
© 2024 Hogrefe Publishing

See p. 213 for instructions on how to obtain the full-sized worksheets as printable PDFs.

Appendix 191

Worksheet 1 (page 5/7)

Guide to a Process-Based Anamnesis

5.3 Behavioral response

Content: what the person did
How did you react?
What did you do more? What was the result of that?
What did you stop doing? What was the result of that?

_____

_____

_____

_____

_____

_____

_____

_____

_____

Processes controlling the way an individual responds behaviorally
Were your actions goal oriented or did you become defensive/avoidant?
Did you become more active (experimenting) or more passive (cautious)?
Were you focusing on a long-term solution or was it more an attempt to endure, persevere, or survive the moment?

_____

_____

_____

_____

_____

_____

_____

_____

_____

This page may be reproduced by the purchaser for personal/clinical use.
From: Michael Svitak and Stefan G. Hofmann: *A Process-Based Approach to CBT* (ISBN 978-0-88937-628-1)
© 2024 Hogrefe Publishing

See p. 213 for instructions on how to obtain the full-sized worksheets as printable PDFs.

192 **Appendix**

Worksheet 1 (page 6/7)

Guide to a Process-Based Anamnesis

5.4 Interactional response

Content: what interactions took place
Did you have or did you attempt to have contact with anyone in this difficult situation? Did anyone respond to the situation and contact you?

_____

_____

_____

_____

_____

_____

_____

_____

_____

Processes dealing with the regulation of interactions/relationships
How did you react interpersonally in the stressful situation?
Did you seek more contact and closeness? Or did you withdraw from others?
Did you ask for help/consolation?
Did you show your difficulties outwardly or did you attempt to hide them?
Did others react to your situation, e.g., offer help? And how did you react to this?

_____

_____

_____

_____

_____

_____

_____

_____

_____

_____

This page may be reproduced by the purchaser for personal/clinical use.
From: Michael Svitak and Stefan G. Hofmann: *A Process-Based Approach to CBT* (ISBN 978-0-88937-628-1)
© 2024 Hogrefe Publishing

See p. 213 for instructions on how to obtain the full-sized worksheets as printable PDFs.

Worksheet 1 (page 7/7)

Guide to a Process-Based Anamnesis

5.5 Somatic/physiological response

Content
What physical reactions did you show or develop? (sleep, tension, pain, appetite)

_____

_____

_____

_____

Process of dealing with physiological responses
How did you react to these physical symptoms?
Did you do anything to influence them? (e.g., medication, doctor visits, resting, taking it easy)
What effect did these actions have? (improvement – no effect – worsening)

_____

_____

_____

_____

6. Consequences of present coping attempts
What positive results have you achieved through your coping attempts so far?
What has become better? What have you prevented?
Do your coping attempts – at least in the short term – have any benefits? (relief, preventing worse, winning time)

_____

_____

_____

_____

What negative effects have resulted? What has become worse?
What's wrong with your current attempts? Why are you seeking help?
What long-term costs are you worried about?

_____

_____

_____

_____

This page may be reproduced by the purchaser for personal/clinical use.
From: Michael Svitak and Stefan G. Hofmann: *A Process-Based Approach to CBT* (ISBN 978-0-88937-628-1)
© 2024 Hogrefe Publishing

See p. 213 for instructions on how to obtain the full-sized worksheets as printable PDFs.

194   **Appendix**

Worksheet 2

Hypothesis Sheet on Relevant Core Processes

Demands/stressors	Vulnerability mechanisms (according to Worksheet 3)	Response mechanisms (according to Worksheet 4)	Consequences
External situation:	Emotional level:	Emotional level:	Short-term consequences:
	Cognitive level:	Cognitive level:	
Internal demand:	Behavioral level:	Behavioral level:	Long-term consequences:
	Interactional level:	Interactional level:	
	Somatic level:	Somatic level:	

Context factors

Protective factors:	Risk factors:

© 2024 Schoen Clinic Bad Staffelstein, Germany. Reprinted with permission.

This page may be reproduced by the purchaser for personal/clinical use.
From: Michael Svitak and Stefan G. Hofmann: *A Process-Based Approach to CBT* (ISBN 978-0-88937-628-1)
© 2024 Hogrefe Publishing

See p. 213 for instructions on how to obtain the full-sized worksheets as printable PDFs.

Appendix   195

Worksheet 3 (page 1/2)

Checklist: Vulnerability Mechanisms

The following checklist identifies empirically supported vulnerability mechanisms that can explain individual differences in coping with demands.

System level	Vulnerability mechanism	No	Suspected	Yes
Neuro-physio-logical level	Ability to regulate tension reduced	☐	☐	☐
	Inhibitory process impaired	☐	☐	☐
	Impaired executive functions	☐	☐	☐
	Disturbed sleep regulation	☐	☐	☐
	Emotion regulation disorder (biological)	☐	☐	☐
Emotional level	**Variations in temperament**			
	Activity level: too high or too low	☐	☐	☐
	Rhythmicity: irregular	☐	☐	☐
	Distractibility: high	☐	☐	☐
	Withdrawal as predominant response	☐	☐	☐
	Adaptability to context: low	☐	☐	☐
	Attention span and persistence: short	☐	☐	☐
	Intensity of reaction: too high or too low	☐	☐	☐
	Threshold of responsiveness: too high or too low	☐	☐	☐
	Negative mood as a trait	☐	☐	☐
	Variations in affective styles			
	Low resilience: reduced stress tolerance	☐	☐	☐
	Negative view of the world	☐	☐	☐
	Impaired ability to decode/interpret nonverbal signals	☐	☐	☐
	Problems decoding internal physical signals	☐	☐	☐
	Difficulties in adapting emotional response to context	☐	☐	☐
	Difficulties in focusing attention	☐	☐	☐
	Specific constructs explaining differences			
	Reduced emotional granularity	☐	☐	☐
	Alexithymia	☐	☐	☐
	Low emotional intelligence	☐	☐	☐

© 2024 Schoen Clinic Bad Staffelstein, Germany. Reprinted with permission.

This page may be reproduced by the purchaser for personal/clinical use.
From: Michael Svitak and Stefan G. Hofmann: *A Process-Based Approach to CBT* (ISBN 978-0-88937-628-1)
© 2024 Hogrefe Publishing

See p. 213 for instructions on how to obtain the full-sized worksheets as printable PDFs.

Appendix

Worksheet 3 (page 2/2)

Checklist: Vulnerability Mechanisms

System level	Vulnerability mechanism	No	Suspected	Yes
Behavioral level	**Variations in learning by associations**			
	Rigid stimulus-response links impair creating new linkages	☐	☐	☐
	Difficulty consolidating newly learned linkages	☐	☐	☐
	Reduced selectivity/differentiation of associations (black and white, all-or-nothing links)	☐	☐	☐
	Overgeneralization tendency of linkages	☐	☐	☐
	Other: _____	☐	☐	☐
	Variations in operant learning			
	Preoperational cognitive level (Piaget)	☐	☐	☐
	High vulnerability for negative reinforcement mechanisms	☐	☐	☐
	Difficulties in reward postponement/impulsivity	☐	☐	☐
	Negative influence due to problematic social learning and model learning	☐	☐	☐
	Deficits in problem-solving skills	☐	☐	☐
Cognitive level	Memory disorders	☐	☐	☐
	Strong tendency to fuse with thoughts	☐	☐	☐
	Inflexible cognitive schemata	☐	☐	☐
	Negative schemata towards self, others, or world	☐	☐	☐
	Attribution bias (e.g., dichotomous, personalizing)	☐	☐	☐
	Negative control beliefs (internal/external)	☐	☐	☐
	Negative problem orientation/problem focus	☐	☐	☐
	Unfavorable metacognitive control (e.g., recursive thinking)	☐	☐	☐
	Unregulated relational learning (e.g., overgeneralizing, jumping to conclusions)	☐	☐	☐
Level of self	Personality disorders	☐	☐	☐
	Negative self-focused attention	☐	☐	☐
	Self-as-content (vs. self-as context)	☐	☐	☐
Relationship level	Attachment disorders	☐	☐	☐
	Difficulty in proximity/distance regulation	☐	☐	☐
	Social skills deficits	☐	☐	☐
Specific constructs	Low regulatory flexibility	☐	☐	☐
	Perfectionism	☐	☐	☐

This page may be reproduced by the purchaser for personal/clinical use.
From: Michael Svitak and Stefan G. Hofmann: *A Process-Based Approach to CBT* (ISBN 978-0-88937-628-1)
© 2024 Hogrefe Publishing

See p. 213 for instructions on how to obtain the full-sized worksheets as printable PDFs.

Appendix   197

Worksheet 4
Checklist: Problematic Response Mechanisms

The following checklist lists empirically supported response mechanisms that can explain individual differences in coping with demands.

System level	Automatic response mechanisms	No	Suspected	Yes
Behavioral core processes	Avoidance and escape behavior	☐	☐	☐
	Safety and reinsurance behavior	☐	☐	☐
	Compulsive behavior	☐	☐	☐
	Generalized experimental avoidance	☐	☐	☐
	Others: _____	☐	☐	☐
Cognitive core processes	Problematic selective attention focus	☐	☐	☐
	Loss of metacognitive control unleashes unregulated cognitive processes	☐	☐	☐
	Cognitive avoidance through thought control	☐	☐	☐
	Cognitive avoidance through thought suppression	☐	☐	☐
	Cognitive avoidance through rumination, brooding and worrying	☐	☐	☐
	Misattribution (internal or external)	☐	☐	☐
	Others: _____	☐	☐	☐
Emotional core processes	Emotion avoidance	☐	☐	☐
	Dysfunctional emotion regulation strategies (e.g., self-harming, drugs and alcohol, eating disorders)	☐	☐	☐
	Others: _____	☐	☐	☐
Motivational core processes	Avoidance motivation	☐	☐	☐
	Situation orientation: difficulty in decision making	☐	☐	☐
	Lack of attachment to one's own values and motives	☐	☐	☐
	Others: _____	☐	☐	☐
Social and interactional core processes	Unfavorable interpersonal response mechanisms (e.g., withdrawal, defensiveness, and prevention of connectedness)	☐	☐	☐
	Neglect of interpersonal resources	☐	☐	☐
	Others: _____	☐	☐	☐

© 2024 Schoen Clinic Bad Staffelstein, Germany. Reprinted with permission.

This page may be reproduced by the purchaser for personal/clinical use.
From: Michael Svitak and Stefan G. Hofmann: *A Process-Based Approach to CBT* (ISBN 978-0-88937-628-1)
© 2024 Hogrefe Publishing

See p. 213 for instructions on how to obtain the full-sized worksheets as printable PDFs.

198 **Appendix**

Worksheet 5

Process-Based Functional Analysis: Support Questions

Triggering situation (S)	Vulnerability (O)	Response (R)		Consequences (C)
		Content	Process	
Selection of a suitable situation **Description of the external situation or trigger (e.g., separation, conflict)**	*List of relevant vulnerability mechanism*	**Cognition** What did you think? **Emotion** What did you feel?	**Cognitive processes** How did you react mentally? How did your thinking change? How long did the change in thinking last? How did you deal with that happening? **Emotional processes** How did you experience your feelings? How did your feelings further evolve? How did you deal with the feelings? Did you try to influence them?	**Short term** What short-term negative or positive consequences did these responses have?
Internal or psychological demands of the situation on the individual (e.g., enduring uncertainty, experiencing intense feelings, dealing with guilt)		**Behavior** What did you do? **Interaction** What happened in your relationship to others? **Physiological reaction** Which physiological reactions did you show?	**Behavioral processes** How did your behavior change? How would you describe your behavior (controlling, avoidance, distraction)? **Interaction processes** How did you respond to the changes in your relationship to others? Has your behavior toward others changed? Have you changed the way you interact? **Physiological processes** How did you respond to the physiological reactions? What did you do to deal with the physical reactions?	**Long term** What long-term negative or positive consequences did these responses have?

© 2024 Schoen Clinic Bad Staffelstein, Germany. Reprinted with permission.

This page may be reproduced by the purchaser for personal/clinical use.
From: Michael Svitak and Stefan G. Hofmann: *A Process-Based Approach to CBT* (ISBN 978-0-88937-628-1)
© 2024 Hogrefe Publishing

See p. 213 for instructions on how to obtain the full-sized worksheets as printable PDFs.

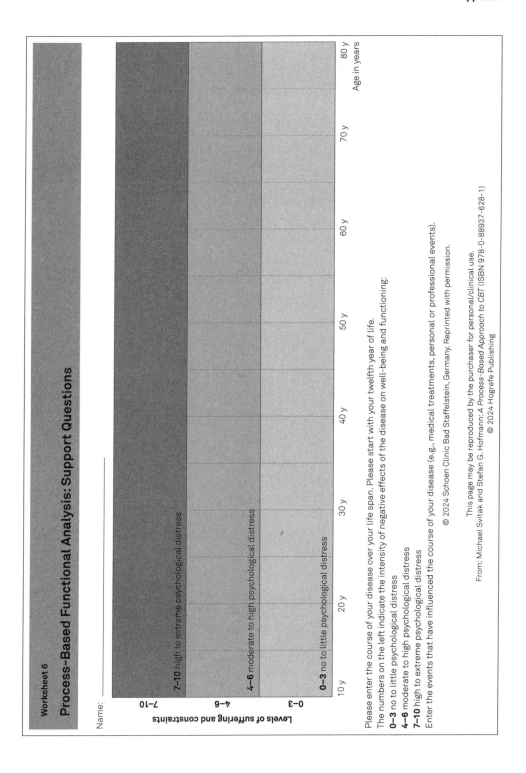

See p. 213 for instructions on how to obtain the full-sized worksheets as printable PDFs.

Worksheet 7

Questions for Relatives About the Development of the Disease

"Thank you for taking the time to support our treatment. I don't want to bother you for long. I care very much about helping <name of patient>. They have told me that your perceptions may help us. Therefore, I would like to ask you a few questions. Any additional clue will help."

1. How do you explain <name>'s mental difficulties?

2. Until when was the world all right from your point of view?

3. How did you first notice that something was wrong?

4. What triggers were apparent to you?

5. How did <name> react? How did they change?

6. Did you notice any changes in behavior?

7. Did <name>'s thought world change?

8. Did <name>'s emotional state change? How did they deal with it?

9. Has their relationship with others changed?

10. What impact does the condition have on you or others around you?

11. What would <name> need to change to cope with the difficulties?

12. Is there anything else you think is important to mention?

13. Specific questions: ...

14. Do you have any questions?

© 2024 Schoen Clinic Bad Staffelstein, Germany. Reprinted with permission.

This page may be reproduced by the purchaser for personal/clinical use.
From: Michael Svitak and Stefan G. Hofmann: *A Process-Based Approach to CBT* (ISBN 978-0-88937-628-1)
© 2024 Hogrefe Publishing

See p. 213 for instructions on how to obtain the full-sized worksheets as printable PDFs.

Appendix 201

Worksheet 8

Process-Based Assessment of Psychopathology

Use the following scale to assess the processes below:

0 = inconspicuous, no disorder
1 = mild disorder/slight abnormalities
2 = moderate disorder/moderate abnormalities
3 = severe disorder/severe abnormalities

	0	1	2	3
Cognitive processes				
Cognitive fusion and lack of distancing from thoughts				
Illusionary, unrealistic processing (lack of context sensitivity)				
Unproductive thinking: circling thoughts, brooding, worrying				
Rigid, automated thought processes				
Dysfunctional attention focus				
Rigid negative view of the world				
Rigid negative image of self				
Harmful or toxic thought processes (e.g., negative self-verbalization)				
Emotional processes				
Emotion regulation disorder: impulsivity or lack of self-soothing				
Impaired emotion perception (e.g., alexithymia)				
Limited expression of feelings (e.g., "false display," i.e., pretending, acting as if)				
Emotion avoidance: suppression, avoidance of emotions				
Low emotional reactivity ("nobody home phenomena")				
Low emotional granularity (low differentiation of feelings)				
Deficits in the use of intrapersonal emotion regulation strategies				
Deficits in the use of interpersonal emotion regulation strategies (e.g., asking for help)				
Self-harming emotion regulation strategies (e.g., self-harm, alcohol)				
Behavioral processes				
Predominantly avoidant behavior control				
Impulsivity and automated behavior control (preoperational, lack of feedback loop)				
Rigid solution attempts without situational adaptation (low context sensitivity)				
Self-harming coping attempts				
Behavioral and problem-solving deficits				
Interactional processes				
Relationship mode: rigid, distrustful, closed, avoidant (vs. flexible, open, trusting)				
Proximity and distance regulation (rigid vs. flexible)				
Lack of social competence skills				
Physiological processes				
Sleep regulation				
Regulation of hunger and satiety				
Tension regulation				

© 2024 Schoen Clinic Bad Staffelstein, Germany. Reprinted with permission.

This page may be reproduced by the purchaser for personal/clinical use.
From: Michael Svitak and Stefan G. Hofmann: *A Process-Based Approach to CBT* (ISBN 978-0-88937-628-1)
© 2024 Hogrefe Publishing

See p. 213 for instructions on how to obtain the full-sized worksheets as printable PDFs.

202 **Appendix**

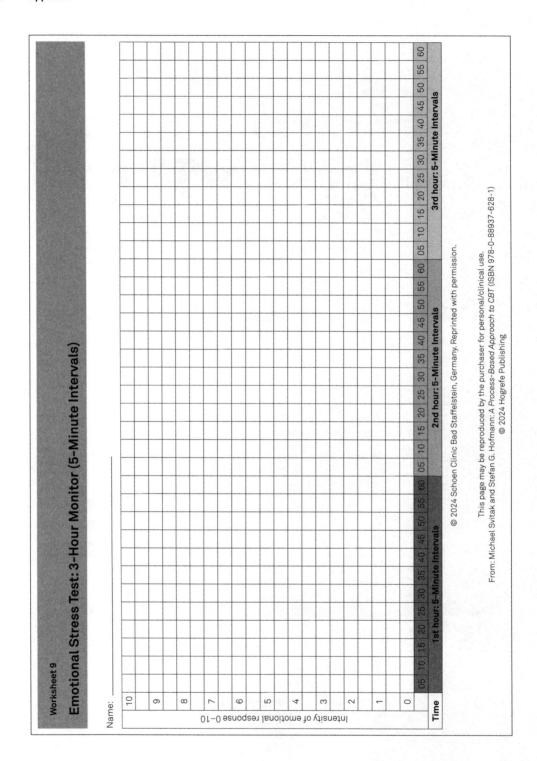

See p. 213 for instructions on how to obtain the full-sized worksheets as printable PDFs.

Appendix 203

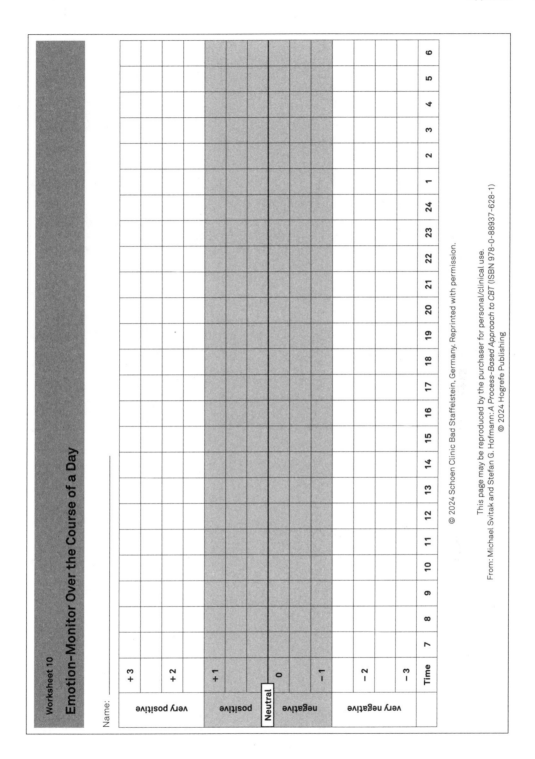

See p. 213 for instructions on how to obtain the full-sized worksheets as printable PDFs.

Worksheet 11

Monitoring Emotions on a Daily Basis

Name: _____

For each hour, please mark the predominant emotional state:
negative affect/negative emotions = red; positive affect/positive emotions = green; neutral = white

Time

Weekday

7	8	9	10	11	12	13	14	15	16	17	18	19	20	21	22	23	24	1	2	3	4	5	6
7	8	9	10	11	12	13	14	15	16	17	18	19	20	21	22	23	24	1	2	3	4	5	6
7	8	9	10	11	12	13	14	15	16	17	18	19	20	21	22	23	24	1	2	3	4	5	6
7	8	9	10	11	12	13	14	15	16	17	18	19	20	21	22	23	24	1	2	3	4	5	6
7	8	9	10	11	12	13	14	15	16	17	18	19	20	21	22	23	24	1	2	3	4	5	6
7	8	9	10	11	12	13	14	15	16	17	18	19	20	21	22	23	24	1	2	3	4	5	6
7	8	9	10	11	12	13	14	15	16	17	18	19	20	21	22	23	24	1	2	3	4	5	6

© 2024 Schoen Clinic Bad Staffelstein, Germany. Reprinted with permission.

This page may be reproduced by the purchaser for personal/clinical use.
From: Michael Svitak and Stefan G. Hofmann: *A Process-Based Approach to CBT* (ISBN 978-0-88937-628-1)
© 2024 Hogrefe Publishing

See p. 213 for instructions on how to obtain the full-sized worksheets as printable PDFs.

See p. 213 for instructions on how to obtain the full-sized worksheets as printable PDFs.

Worksheet 12

24/7 Monitor

Name: _____

Monitor: _____

For each hour, please mark by shading the box, whether the symptom you are monitoring was – to a relevant degree – present.

Weekday | | | | | | | | | | **Time**

Weekday	7	8	9	10	11	12	13	14	15	16	17	18	19	20	21	22	23	24	1	2	3	4	5	6
_____	7	8	9	10	11	12	13	14	15	16	17	18	19	20	21	22	23	24	1	2	3	4	5	6
_____	7	8	9	10	11	12	13	14	15	16	17	18	19	20	21	22	23	24	1	2	3	4	5	6
_____	7	8	9	10	11	12	13	14	15	16	17	18	19	20	21	22	23	24	1	2	3	4	5	6
_____	7	8	9	10	11	12	13	14	15	16	17	18	19	20	21	22	23	24	1	2	3	4	5	6
_____	7	8	9	10	11	12	13	14	15	16	17	18	19	20	21	22	23	24	1	2	3	4	5	6
_____	7	8	9	10	11	12	13	14	15	16	17	18	19	20	21	22	23	24	1	2	3	4	5	6
_____	7	8	9	10	11	12	13	14	15	16	17	18	19	20	21	22	23	24	1	2	3	4	5	6

Appendix

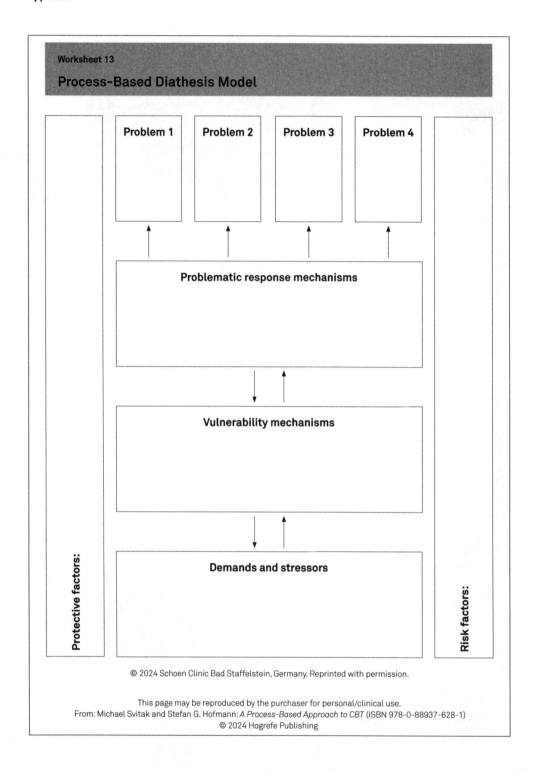

See p. 213 for instructions on how to obtain the full-sized worksheets as printable PDFs.

Worksheet 14

Evaluating Adaptivity Through the Extended Evolutionary Metamodel

		Variation	Selection	Retention	Context
Dimensions	Emotion				
	Cognition				
	Attention				
	Self				
	Overt behavior				
	Motivation				
Levels	Biophysiological				
	Sociocultural				

© 2024 Schoen Clinic Bad Staffelstein, Germany. Reprinted with permission by Stefan G. Hofmann.

This page may be reproduced by the purchaser for personal/clinical use.
From: Michael Svitak and Stefan G. Hofmann: *A Process-Based Approach to CBT* (ISBN 978-0-88937-628-1)
© 2024 Hogrefe Publishing

See p. 213 for instructions on how to obtain the full-sized worksheets as printable PDFs.

208 **Appendix**

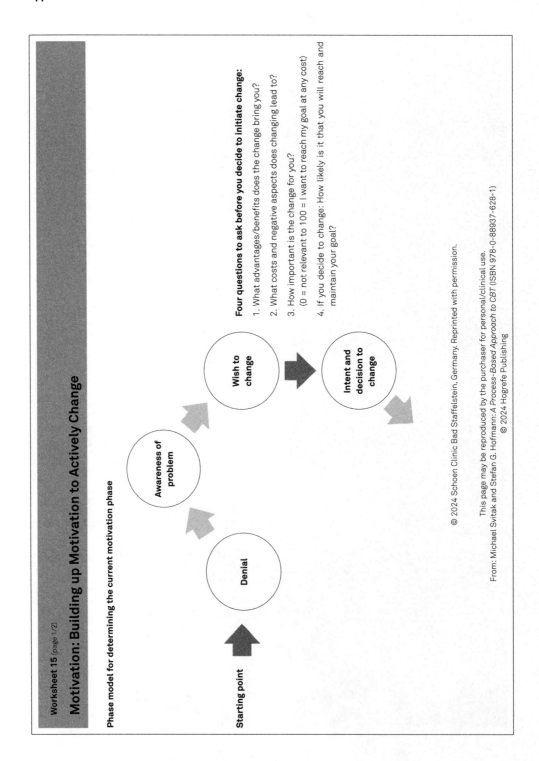

See p. 213 for instructions on how to obtain the full-sized worksheets as printable PDFs.

Worksheet 15 (page 2/2)

Motivation to Change

Four ingredients for a robust decision to change
What is the specific change target?

---

1. The desired change must bring important advantages for me

What do I hope to achieve through the change? What do I long for? What will I have more of? What will I leave behind?

Therapist rating: Are the desired advantages of change convincing enough?
(not convincing) 0 – 25 – 50 – 75 – 100 *(strongly convincing)*

2. I must be willing to tolerate the costs/disadvantages of the change

What are the disadvantages of the change (why I have not done it so far)? What commitment am I willing to make for it?

Therapist rating: Is the willingness and commitment convincing enough?
(not convincing) 0 – 25 – 50 – 75 – 100 *(strongly convincing)*

3. The desired change must be really important for me

Explain why it is important to you to achieve your therapy goal. On a scale of 0 to 100, how important is the goal to your life?

Therapist rating: Is the perceived importance to change convincing enough?
(not convincing) 0 – 25 – 50 – 75 – 100 *(strongly convincing)*

4. I must be convinced that I can somehow achieve and maintain the goal

How confident are you that you can make the change happen? What can you do to influence the probability of success? How likely are you to succeed (0% to 100%)?

Therapist rating: Is the positive outcome expectancy convincing enough?
(not convincing) 0 – 25 – 50 – 75 – 100 *(strongly convincing)*

© 2024 Schoen Clinic Bad Staffelstein, Germany. Reprinted with permission.

This page may be reproduced by the purchaser for personal/clinical use.
From: Michael Svitak and Stefan G. Hofmann: *A Process-Based Approach to CBT* (ISBN 978-0-88937-628-1)
© 2024 Hogrefe Publishing

See p. 213 for instructions on how to obtain the full-sized worksheets as printable PDFs.

Appendix

Worksheet 16

Cost-Benefit Analysis for Treatment

	Advantages/benefits	Disadvantages/costs
Previous handling of the situation/ demands	What desired effect is achieved by the current handling?	What is the problem with your current handling of the situation?
	What negative effects are currently being prevented?	What are the disadvantages in the long run?
	What other benefits does the status quo have?	What new problems does it create?
Anticipated handling of demands/ stressors with the help of therapy	What are you hoping for through achieving your therapy goals?	What disadvantages of change do you see?
	What desired effects would it have?	What new difficulties/obstacles may arise?
	What is the main benefit you are hoping for?	What can go wrong? What are you afraid of?
		What do I have to deal with then?

© 2024 Schoen Clinic Bad Staffelstein, Germany. Reprinted with permission.

This page may be reproduced by the purchaser for personal/clinical use.
From: Michael Svitak and Stefan G. Hofmann: *A Process-Based Approach to CBT* (ISBN 978-0-88937-628-1)
© 2024 Hogrefe Publishing

See p. 213 for instructions on how to obtain the full-sized worksheets as printable PDFs.

Appendix 211

Worksheet 17

Evidence-Based Treatment Strategies (based on Kazantzis et al., 2018)

System level	Effective strategies
Treatment processes (change processes)	
Cognitive processes	• Decentering (e.g., defusion, mindfulness, detached mindfulness) • Attention focus
Cognition	• Cognitive reappraisal • Reframing • Increasing self-efficacy • Establishing positive outcome expectancies
Behavior	• Confrontation • Behavioral activation
Emotion	• Acceptance
Motivation	• Goal setting • Values
In-session processes (therapeutic interactions)	
	• Therapeutic relationship (alliance) • Goal consensus and collaboration • Feedback • Homework

© 2024 Schoen Clinic Bad Staffelstein, Germany.

This page may be reproduced by the purchaser for personal/clinical use.
From: Michael Svitak and Stefan G. Hofmann: *A Process-Based Approach to CBT* (ISBN 978-0-88937-628-1)
© 2024 Hogrefe Publishing

See p. 213 for instructions on how to obtain the full-sized worksheets as printable PDFs.

Appendix

Worksheet 18

Standard Psychotherapeutic Procedures for Targeted Interventions

The standard procedures listed here are in accordance with the training standards of the Inter-organizational Task Force on Cognitive and Behavioral Psychology Doctoral Education (Klepac et al., 2012).

Core processes of psychopathology	Psychotherapeutic standard procedures
Physiological regulation processes	• Relaxation and tension reduction techniques
Behavioral processes	• Contingence management • Stimulus-control techniques • Shaping • Self-management techniques • Exposition therapies • Behavior activation • Behavioral trainings
Emotion regulation processes	• Coping and emotion regulation (including exposition therapy) • Acceptance
Cognitive processes	• Problem solving • Attention focusing and directing techniques • Cognitive reappraisal • Modification of core beliefs • Defusion • Value clarification
Social and interpersonal processes	• Interpersonal skills training
Multidimensional constructs	• Mindfulness training • Motivational techniques • Crisis management und suicidality management

© 2024 Schoen Clinic Bad Staffelstein, Germany. Reprinted with permission.

This page may be reproduced by the purchaser for personal/clinical use.
From: Michael Svitak and Stefan G. Hofmann: *A Process-Based Approach to CBT* (ISBN 978-0-88937-628-1)
© 2024 Hogrefe Publishing

See p. 213 for instructions on how to obtain the full-sized worksheets as printable PDFs.

Notes on Supplementary Materials

The following materials for your book can be downloaded free of charge once you register on the Hogrefe website:

Appendix: Tools and Resources

Worksheets 1–18
Worksheet 1:   Guide to a Process-Based Anamnesis
Worksheet 2:   Hypothesis Sheet on Relevant Core Processes
Worksheet 3:   Checklist: Vulnerability Mechanisms
Worksheet 4:   Checklist: Problematic Response Mechanisms
Worksheet 5:   Process-Based Functional Analysis: Support Questions
Worksheet 6:   Process-Based Functional Analysis: Support Questions
Worksheet 7:   Questions for Relatives About the Development of the Disease
Worksheet 8:   Process-Based Assessment of Psychopathology
Worksheet 9:   Emotional Stress Test: 3-Hour Monitor (5-Minute Intervals)
Worksheet 10: Emotion-Monitor Over the Course of a Day
Worksheet 11: Monitoring Emotions on a Daily Basis
Worksheet 12: 24/7 Monitor
Worksheet 13: Process-Based Diathesis Model
Worksheet 14: Evaluating Adaptivity Through the Extended Evolutionary Metamodel
Worksheet 15: Motivation: Building up Motivation to Actively Change
Worksheet 16: Cost-Benefit Analysis for Treatment
Worksheet 17: Evidence-Based Treatment Strategies (based on Kazantzis et al., 2018)
Worksheet 18: Standard Psychotherapeutic Procedures for Targeted Interventions

How to proceed:
1. Go to www.hgf.io/media and create a user account. If you already have one, please log in.

2. Go to **My supplementary materials** in your account dashboard and enter the code below. You will automatically be redirected to the download area, where you can access and download the supplementary materials.

Code: **B-ELWRLI**

To make sure you have permanent direct access to all the materials, we recommend that you download them and save them on your device.

Peer Commentaries

Many clinicians and clinical scientists around the world have heard of the important innovation referred to as 'a process-based approach to CBT', but in my experience many of those individuals are not quite sure what it is or why it's important. Now, all answers covering both theory and practice are clearly laid out in this well-written illustration of this approach. All clinicians and therapists should take advantage of this volume to understand the basic principles of dealing with underlying behavioral and affective processes rather than symptoms in their attempts to relieve human suffering associated with psychopathology.

David H. Barlow, PhD, ABPP, Professor Emeritus of Psychology and Psychiatry and the Founder of Center for Anxiety and Related Disorders, Boston University, MA

There is a race afoot for the leading theoretical position in CBT and it's being won by those advocating a process-based approach. The disease model has dominated clinical diagnosis, but it has failed to reflect the reality that 80% of 'disorders' are comorbid with other 'disorders'. This work is an excellent introduction to the rationale, conceptualization, and treatment implications of a process-based therapy. It is concise, powerful, and clear, and will give the reader the understanding and the tools to transcend the fictionalized world of the current diagnostic manual. I highly recommend this excellent book.

Robert L. Leahy, PhD, Director of the American Institute for Cognitive Therapy, New York City, NY

This book is like an eye-opener to the vision of future psychotherapy. Highly integrative and still evidence-based, dynamic case formulations instead of inflexible school-based problem definitions, and open for continuous developments: Psychotherapy overcomes the barriers of traditional thinking, and embraces the complexity and individuality of clinical problems.

Winfried Rief, PhD, Spokesperson of the LOEWE Center DYNAMIC and Head of the Department of Clinical Psychology and Psychotherapy, University of Marburg, Germany

New edition of this effective toolbox for treating trauma survivors is even more comprehensive

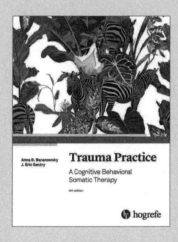

4th ed. 2023, xii + 228 pp.,
$59.00 / € 50.95
ISBN 978-0-88937-592-5
Also available as eBook

Anna B. Baranowsky / J. Eric Gentry

Trauma Practice
A Cognitive Behavioral Somatic Therapy

This popular, practical resource for clinicians caring for trauma survivors has been fully updated and expanded. It remains a key toolkit of cognitive behavioral somatic therapy (CBST) techniques for clinicians who want to enhance their skills in treating trauma. Baranowsky and Gentry help practitioners find the right tools to guide trauma survivors toward growth and healing. Reinforcing this powerful intervention is the addition of a deeper emphasis on the preparatory phase for therapists, including the therapists' own ability to self-regulate their autonomic system during client encounters.

Throughout the acclaimed book, an effective tri-phasic model for trauma treatment is constructed (safety and stabilization; working through trauma; reconnection with a meaningful life) as guiding principle, enabling a phased delivery that is fitted to the survivor's relational and processing style. The authors present, clearly and in detail, an array of techniques, protocols, and interventions for treating trauma survivors (cognitive, behavioral, somatic, and emotional/relational). These include popular and effective CBST techniques, approaches inspired by research on neuroplasticity, and interventions informed by polyvagal theory. Many techniques include links to video or audio material demonstrating how to carry-out the intervention. Further sections are devoted to forward-facing trauma therapy, a safe, effective, and accelerated method of treating trauma, and to clinician self-care. Handouts for clients are also available for download.

www.hogrefe.com

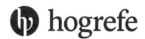

Positive CBT focusing on building what's right, not on reducing what is wrong

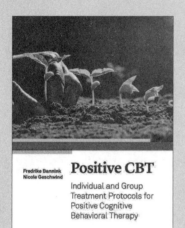

2021, viii + 144 pages incl. online materials
US $49.80 / € 34.95
ISBN 978-0-88937-578-9
Also available as eBook

Fredrike Bannink / Nicole Geschwind

Positive CBT

Individual and Group Treatment Protocols for Positive Cognitive Behavioral Therapy

Positive CBT integrates positive psychology and solution-focused brief therapy within a cognitive-behavioral framework. It focuses not on reducing what is wrong, but on building what is right. This fourth wave CBT, developed by Fredrike Bannink, is now being applied worldwide for various psychological disorders. After an introductory chapter exploring the three approaches incorporated in positive CBT, the research into the individual treatment protocol for use with clients with depression by Nicole Geschwind and her colleagues at Maastricht University is presented.

The two 8-session treatment protocols provide practitioners with a step-by-step guide on how to apply positive CBT with individual clients and groups. This approach goes beyond symptom reduction and instead focuses on the client's desired future, on finding exceptions to problems and identifying competencies. Topics such as self-compassion, optimism, gratitude, and behavior maintenance are explored.

In addition to the protocols, two workbooks for clients are available online for practitioners. They can be downloaded from the Hogrefe website after registration.

www.hogrefe.com

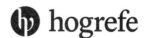

Advances in Psychotherapy – Evidence-Based Practice

Developed and edited with the support of the Society of Clinical Psychology (APA Division 12)

Editor-in-chief
Danny Wedding, PhD, MPH

Associate editors
Jonathan S. Comer, PhD
Linda Carter Sobell, PhD, ABPP
Kenneth E. Freedland, PhD
J. Kim Penberthy, PhD, ABPP

- *Practice-oriented*
- *Evidence-based*
- *Expert authors*
- *Easy-to-read*
- *Compact*
- *Cost-effective*

Latest releases

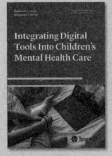
Integrating Digital Tools Into Children's Mental Health Care
Volume 52

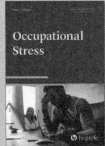
Occupational Stress
Volume 51

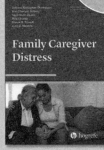
Family Caregiver Distress
Volume 50

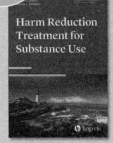
Harm Reduction Treatment for Substance Use
Volume 49

www.hogrefe.com/apt

hogrefe

Advances in Psychotherapy – Evidence-Based Practice

All volumes of the series at a glance

Affirmative Counseling for Transgender and Gender Diverse Clients (Vol. 45)
Alcohol Use Disorders (Vol. 10)
Alzheimer's Disease and Dementia (Vol. 38)
ADHD in Adults, 2nd ed., (Vol. 35)
ADHD in Children and Adolescents, 2nd. ed., (Vol. 33)
Autism Spectrum Disorder (Vol. 29)
Binge Drinking and Alcohol Misuse Among College Students and Young Adults (Vol. 32)
Bipolar Disorder (Vol. 1, 2nd ed.)
Body Dysmorphic Disorder (Vol. 44)
Childhood Maltreatment (Vol. 4, 2nd ed.)
Childhood Obesity (Vol. 39)
Chronic Illness in Children and Adolescents (Vol. 9)
Chronic Pain (Vol. 11)
Depression (Vol. 18)
Eating Disorders (Vol. 13)
Elimination Disorders in Children and Adolescents (Vol. 16)
Family Caregiver Distress (Vol. 50)
Generalized Anxiety Disorder (Vol. 24)
Growing Up with Domestic Violence (Vol. 23)
Harm Reduction Treatment for Substance Use (Vol. 49)
Headache (Vol. 30)
Heart Disease (Vol. 2)
Hoarding Disorder (Vol. 40)
Hypochondriasis and Health Anxiety (Vol. 19)
Insomnia (Vol. 42)
Integrating Digital Tools into Children's Mental Health Care (Vol. 52)
Internet Addiction (Vol. 41)
Language Disorders in Children and Adolescents (Vol. 28)
Mindfulness (Vol. 37)
Multiple Sclerosis (Vol. 36)
Nicotine and Tobacco Dependence (Vol. 21)
Nonsuicidal Self-Injury (Vol. 22)
Obsessive-Compulsive Disorder in Adults (Vol. 31)
Occupational Stress (Vol. 51)
Persistent Depressive Disorders (Vol. 43)
Phobic and Anxiety Disorders in Children and Adolescents (Vol. 27)
Problem and Pathological Gambling (Vol. 8)
Psychological Approaches to Cancer Care (Vol. 46)
Public Health Tools for Practicing Psychologists (Vol. 20)
Sexual Dysfunction in Women (Vol. 25)
Sexual Dysfunction in Men (Vol. 26)
Sexual Violence (Vol. 17)
Social Anxiety Disorder (Vol. 12)
Substance Use Problems (Vol. 15, 2nd ed.)
Suicidal Behavior (Vol. 14, 2nd ed.)
The Schizophrenia Spectrum (Vol. 5, 2nd ed.)
Time-Out in Child Behavior Management (Vol. 48)
Treating Victims of Mass Disaster and Terrorism (Vol. 6)
Women and Drinking: Preventing Alcohol-Exposed Pregnancies (Vol. 34)

Prices: US $29.80 / € 24.95 per volume. Standing order price US $24.80 / € 19.95 per volume (minimum 4 successive volumes) + postage & handling. Special rates for APA Division 12 and Division 42 members

www.hogrefe.com/apt

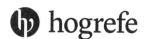